breathing
works
for
asthma

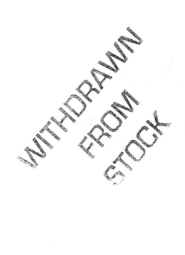

Dr Mike Thomas is the GPIAG Clinical Research Fellow with the Department of General Practice and Primary Care, University of Aberdeen and works principally in the field of respiratory research and education. He continues to work part-time in general practice, and is also Primary Care Advisor to Gloucestershire NHS Research and Development Support Unit, a specialist advisor to the UK National Asthma Campaign. He has published original asthma research, including recent papers in the *British Medical Journal* and *Thorax* on the overlap between asthma and abnormal breathing patterns, and leads an ongoing multi-disciplinary research team investigating the effectiveness of breathing exercises in asthma.

breathing
works
for
asthma

Dinah Bradley
DIP PHYS, MNZSP, NZRP

Tania Clifton-Smith
DIP PHYS, MNZSP, NZMTA, NZRP

Foreword by Dr Mike Thomas

Kyle Cathie Limited

First published in Great Britain 2003 by
Kyle Cathie Limited
122 Arlington Road
London NW1 7HP
general.enquiries@kyle-cathie.com
www.kylecathie.com

First published in New Zealand in 2002 by
Tandem Press

2 4 6 8 10 9 7 5 3 1

ISBN 1 85626 494 7

Senior Editor: Muna Reyal
Cover design: Mark Latter at Vivid Design
Text design: Robert Updegraff
Production: Sha Huxtable
Printed and bound in Great Britain by Biddles Ltd, Guildford

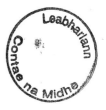

Contents

Acknowledgements

To Helen Benton and Bob Ross, heartfelt appreciation and thanks for publishing our book, and to Jane Hingston for helpful and constructive editing management.

To Dr Allen Liang for his generous support of this project.

To Dr Mike Thomas for his foreword.

To the Asthma and Respiratory Foundation of New Zealand (Inc.) for use of Asthma Education material.

To the Auckland Asthma Society.

To our families and friends for their love and… endurance.

Last but not least – the kind contribution of illuminating comments from people who live with asthma. Many thanks to you all.

Foreword

It is with great pleasure that I write the foreword to the UK edition of this useful
and comprehensive book on healthy breathing techniques in asthma, written
by Dinah Bradley and Tania Clifton-Smith. The authors are both practising
respiratory physiotherapists with great hands-on and theoretical experience in
the diagnosis and treatment of breathing disorders in asthma. They are well
known in professional and public circles for their work and for their writing, and
have done much to further interest in breathing exercises for the management
of asthma in the general public and amongst fellow professionals. This book is
the fruit of their background knowledge and practical experience, and is a very
useful introduction to breathing exercises to the interested lay reader as well
as being a valuable source of general scientific information on asthma. The
authors have managed to combine pragmatic and easy-to-understand
practical advice with a well-presented and readable summary of the important
physiological principles underlying asthma and the breathing disorders that
may be associated with it. They show how it is possible to improve symptoms
and quality of life for people with asthma by practising simple exercises and
they explain how these exercises may work. The frequent quotes from patients
they have treated and helped to gain control of their asthma symptoms
correspond very much with my own experience of diagnosing, treating and
researching this area over the last 10 years.

Asthma has been described as the epidemic of our time, and the
prevalence of asthma in the general public has trebled within a single lifetime,
particularly amongst children. For reasons that we do not fully understand, we
are becoming more allergic and wheezier. This is a pattern that is seen all
around the developed world in association with Westernised lifestyles, and has
been described as a disease of affluence. Scientists are slowly unravelling the
complex reasons behind this notable phenomenon, and we all live in the hope
that prevention will become possible within our times. In the meantime,

however, asthma remains a reality for many millions of people. Although we have many treatments for asthma, we do not have a cure, and many people need to take regular medication to control their asthma on a long-term basis. In spite of very effective treatment to prevent asthma attacks and symptoms and to treat them when they do occur, surveys reveal that many people still have very significant symptoms from asthma, and for many people asthma impairs their quality of life and limits their horizons[1;2]. It is also clear that in spite of evidence of effectiveness and safety, many people do not like having to use medication on a regular basis to control their asthma. They resent being tied to their inhalers, worry that the effects will wear off over time and are concerned about the side effects of long-term treatment.

There is great public and increasing professional interest in non-drug treatments for asthma, with evidence in the UK that one third of people with asthma use Complementary and Alternative Medicine (CAM) to treat their asthma, usually in addition to, but sometimes instead of, standard medical treatment[3]. Breathing exercises and yoga have been widely used to treat asthma in Eastern and Western societies for many years, and generally centre on manipulating the respiratory pattern to reduce respiratory frequency and hyperventilation. As explained in this book, breathing is a complex action, involving many muscle groups and controlled by different parts of the brain. Although unconscious reflexes control basic breathing patterns, we can modify natural patterns if we consciously decide to, and sometimes natural patterns of breathing may become altered through a variety of physical and psychological mechanisms, and dysfunctional 'bad' breathing patterns may occur. Can these patterns be corrected by breathing retraining? Unfortunately, in contrast to the wealth of high-quality evidence from scientific studies on drug-based treatment in asthma, often driven by the pharmaceutical industry, there is a paucity of information on non-pharmacological treatments, such as breathing retraining. A review of the scientific studies on breathing exercises for asthma in the 'evidence based' Cochrane Library concluded that while there were suggestions that such treatment was effective, too few rigorous studies have been to make firm conclusions[4], and calls for more research. As part of a collaborative research group that includes the University of Aberdeen,

University of Leicester and the NHS Gloucestershire Research and Development Support Unit, I have investigated this area and our recent work has shown that there may indeed be a major overlap between asthma and abnormal, dysfunctional breathing. We have recently published papers showing that up to one in three people with asthma have evidence of abnormal breathing[5], and that a physiotherapy-based breathing retraining programme can improve their symptoms and quality of life[6]. Further studies to confirm these findings and investigate the way in which breathing retraining works are currently underway.

The accusation is sometimes levelled against doctors that they are too focused on pharmacological 'drug-based' treatments for illnesses, and it may be that there is some truth in this in the asthma field. Doctors are encouraged to be sceptical of claims of effective treatment, drug based or otherwise, until that treatment has been proven to be effective in properly conducted trials. The shortage of such evidence has meant that breathing therapy has often not been part of mainstream practice, and so has not been available to many people. We are, however, starting to see more interest and more trials done in CAM and in breathing retraining in asthma. Doctors and scientists are perhaps slowly catching up with what therapists like Dinah and Tania, and their patients, have known for some time – that many people with asthma breathe badly and that with a little time and effort, something can be done to correct this. I would fully concur with their advice that this is time and effort well spent! I have seen patients many times who have been found to have abnormal 'dysfunctional' breathing as a factor in their asthma, and who have come back after breathing treatment similar to that described in this book feeling so much better, feeling 'in control' and understanding themselves and their bodies better. I hope that you, like me, will find this book useful, stimulating, educational and enjoyable.

Dr Mike Thomas
GPIAG Research Fellow,
Department of General Practice
University of Aberdeen

References

1. Price D, Ryan D, Pearce L, Bride F. The AIR study: asthma in real life. *Asthma J* 1999;**4**:74–8.

2. Rabe KF, Vermeire PA, Soriano JB, Maier WC. Clinical management of asthma in 1999: the Asthma Insights and Reality in Europe (AIRE) study. *Eur Respir J* 2000;**16**:802–7.

3. Ernst E. Complementary therapies for asthma: what patients use. *J Asthma* 1998;**35**:667–71.

4. Holloway E and Ram FSF. Breathing exercises for asthma (Cochrane review). The Cochrane Library Issue 3. 2000. Oxford, Update Software.

5. Thomas M, McKinley RK, Freeman E, Foy C. Prevalence of dysfunctional breathing in patients treated for asthma in Primary Care: a cross-sectional survey. *BMJ* 2001; **322**:1098–100.

6. Thomas M, McKinley RK, Freeman E, Foy C, Prodger P, Price D. Breathing retraining for dysfunctional breathing in asthma – a randomised controlled trial. *Thorax* 2003;**58**:110–5.

Introduction

Asthma is a fascinating subject. Millions of people worldwide suffer from its symptoms – with mild to life-threatening episodes. A recent World Health Organization report states that 150 million people have this disorder; it affects people of all ages, all races 'humble or poor, rich or renowned'. It has even been observed in animals. Yet ask five different medical specialists what the causes are and you'll get five different answers. Similarly, asking five alternative health practitioners the same question will reveal the same diversity of opinion.

There have been hundreds upon thousands of books written on this mysterious, breathing-related disease, from orthodox sources through to alternative 'cures'. Research articles and latest findings are all freely available from numerous websites. Often patients know more about what's new than their overworked doctors.

At Breathing Works, our Auckland-based Breathing Pattern Disorders/Hyperventilation Syndromes Clinics (the first independent service of this kind in Australasia) we see many people, referred for help with their asthma education and management. We are registered practising physiotherapists and we have both published books and presented papers on Breathing Pattern Disorders nationally and internationally. Why do we think we have anything extra to add?

There are two reasons: the first is that people with asthma often develop truly dreadful breathing patterns. They use their chest muscles the wrong way, they breathe through their mouths, and they breathe too fast. We see this all the time in our clinics. There are many reasons why this happens and we will cover them in this book. Our concern is that these 'bad breathing' patterns can make asthma worse, even triggering attacks – or to use the more politically correct term, episodes. Curiously, since the advent of user-friendly inhalers thirty-odd years ago and newer asthma 'wonder drugs', less attention has been paid by the medical profession to the business of breathing itself.

Asthma awareness and education programmes highlight information about what goes on inside the chest – what happens to the airways, how to use the various devices for delivering asthma medications, how to reduce environmental triggers. But we want to add to this information. We want to show those with asthma the value of physical coping skills – i.e. learning what's happening on the outside of the chest wall and including this as a vital part of asthma self-management.

Knowing how to breathe properly and efficiently by employing physical coping skills enhances drug therapies, and in many instances helps people reduce medications, and their stress levels, and to exercise more enjoyably.

The second reason is that we believe you can breathe too much. Using the wrong combination of chest muscles leads to chronic over-breathing or hyperventilation. This in itself is stressful to both body and soul, and is a disorder people can do without, whether they have asthma or not. Over-breathing causes unpleasant and alarming symptoms which tend to be lumped together with the symptoms of airway hyper-reactivity (asthma). Two disorders for the price of one!

Newly diagnosed asthmatics are likely to be bamboozled by conflicting information and views on the right and wrong ways to manage their symptoms. Parents of young children with asthma report that problems in dealing with their own anxieties (and over-breathing) are compounded when they are faced with differences of opinion. This of course leads to more stress.

We at Breathing Works challenge everyone who has asthma to take responsibility for their own breathing, and aim for the best, mechanically efficient, physiologically correct breathing.

Make balanced breathing your starting point, and give any of the choices you subsequently take in managing your own asthma the very best start, from a strong foundation based on tiptop, dynamic, calm, beautiful breathing.

Dinah Bradley & Tania Clifton-Smith

CHAPTER 1

Breathe well to be well

I have had asthma all my life. As a child my breathing was so bad that sometimes I would cough continuously through the night. My parents set up a bed for me in the lounge because if I slept in one of the bedrooms I kept the entire household awake! I was always tired. Even though my asthma was quite well managed I know I was over-reliant on my inhalers – simple pleasures such as a walk in the country would set me off. Asthma was a large part of my life, but I was one of many who just accepted it and lived with it. Three years ago I lost my voice again and as a trainer for a busy company this was pretty serious for me. My GP at the time had tried everything and suggested I visit Breathing Works for an assessment: I am now in control – I only get exercise-induced asthma and I am a brilliant nose-diaphragm breather. All I can say is how amazing it was to be shown proper breathing. **Teresa, 33**

Asthma is a word that comes from ancient Greek; it means 'difficult breathing' or 'panting'. Originally asthma included all breathing problems but was redefined in the twentieth century as 'difficulty breathing due to a problem that begins in the bronchial tubes of the lungs'. The bronchial tubes become over-sensitive and react to things that don't affect other people. These things are called triggers. The triggers cause the airways to swell inside, become inflamed and make more mucus. This causes the muscle in the airway to tighten. All of this means that it is much harder to breathe in and out. You may feel short of breath, tight in the chest, wheezy (your breath might 'whistle' in and out) or you might have a cough. There are many triggers: exercise, emotional stress, chest infections, sinus infections, colds, flu, air pollutants, certain drugs, chemicals, tobacco smoke, weather conditions, allergies (the most common allergens are dust mites, moulds, animal fur, feathers and cockroaches), fragrances and ***poor breathing patterns***. Poor breathing patterns can also enhance your reaction and sensitivity to any of the above triggers.

Good breathing patterns are vital to good health. When we look at the structure and mechanics of the body we see it is designed so that we breathe using our nose in conjunction with the power of a muscle called the diaphragm. The diaphragm draws air into the lungs as easily as a syringe draws up fluid.

When we talk about breathing muscles we refer to primary and accessory muscles. The primary muscles are the number one muscles used all the time, while accessory muscles are those called upon in certain situations – but they are certainly not designed to work all the time.

The diaphragm, the main primary muscle, is responsible for 70–80 per cent of the work during quiet breathing; the remaining 20–30 per cent is carried out by neck and shoulder muscles that are attached to the ribcage. Chapter 5 looks at these in more detail.

The mechanics of breathing

During inhalation the diaphragm muscle brings down the powerful central tendon, which increases the vertical diameter of the chest cage. This movement is opposed by the bony limitations of the chest but also especially by the resistance of the abdominal contents contained in the abdominal girdle. The abdominal girdle is made up of abdominal muscles; it is important that these are also in tiptop shape. Chapter 10 shows us how.

The twelve ribs attached to the spine and chest-bone spin in their joints and stretch with the cartilage, allowing the outwards and upwards action of the ribcage to occur. This same action micro-massages the joints of the spine, maintaining flexibility and health of the joints like a well-greased hinge. The diaphragm and the ribcage co-ordinate to move downwards, outwards and then upwards – an action similar to raising the handle on a bucket.

This action creates pressure changes within the thoracic cage, causing the lungs to fill with air somewhat like a piano accordion that is stretched and compressed to create varying sounds. For the volume to increase the chest will expand and move in three different directions. The greatest increase will occur when all three vertical, transverse and anterior-posterior movements occur together. This combination of movement is commonly used in high-energy-demanding situations such as running.

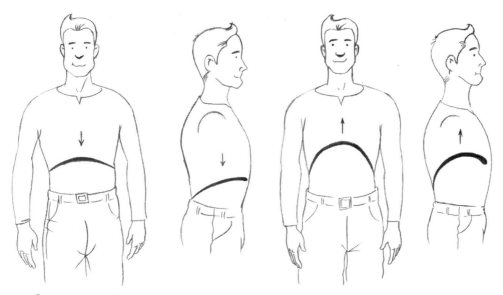

On the in-breath the diaphragm flattens. On the out-breath the diaphragm rises.

The air you inhale is about 21 per cent oxygen; this travels in through your nose, and then passes into the trachea (the main windpipe), after having passed through the pharynx and larynx. The air then travels through the bronchial tubes into bronchioles and to the alveoli, where the exchange of gases occurs, i.e. of oxygen and carbon dioxide.

The musculo-skeletal structures surrounding the lungs relax, assisting the lungs to deflate and exhale the air. During breathing under load the abdominal muscles are called upon to help with forced exhalation. The air you exhale contains carbon dioxide, which is the end result of this process.

Although it appears quite simple the process of breathing requires a lot of energy and co-ordination.

Why breathe well?

Breathing is hard-wired from birth – nose, belly, rhythmical and flowing. It is one of the things parents look for, listen to and use as a tool to guide them on the wellbeing of their children.

Babies spend long periods suckling, which would be impossible if they had to pause to draw breath all the time. They breathe at a rate of perhaps 50 breaths per minute; this changes to 15–25 breaths as a child; and finally as an adult we should be breathing 10–14 breaths a minute at rest.

Nose-belly breathing is the pattern we are designed to maintain at rest (and during light-to-moderate activity – depending on fitness levels) throughout life. But for many children and adults this pattern has been lost for a variety of both physical and emotional reasons (see Chapter 2 as to why and how).

Control of breathing

Breathing is controlled by the respiratory centre in the brain. It mainly works on automatic control from feedback from nerves in the lungs, muscles and the carbon dioxide levels in the blood. It is remarkable in that it is under both voluntary and involuntary control.

We can control our breathing at a conscious level – for example when we learn to play a wind instrument we alter our breathing pattern. Think about it: you can change your breathing if you feel like it. Don't worry that you will stop – the drive to breathe will always prevail.

The benefits of good breathing patterns

- Postural stability: Creating a mobile, supportive spine that leads to correct posture, fluid movement, agility and correct locomotion.
- Good spinal health leads to the good health of the nervous system (which is housed in the spine), allowing us to remain in a physiologically and emotionally balanced state.
- Good breathing maintains good lung pressures for energy-efficient breathing.
- Good breathing ensures oxygenation of the lower lobes of the lungs which have a rich blood supply.
- Voice production: Our voice is the result of the breath flowing over the vocal folds (formerly known as vocal cords). Good diaphragm (belly) breathing gives us an easy, flowing breath, creating good pitch and voice control. Upper chest-breathing can give us a gaspy, higher-pitched voice. The state of the voice can assist as a warning sign for parents with children who have asthma, as voice change is a sign of tightened airways or poor breathing patterns.

- Removal of waste products: Breathing is one of the most important ways for the body to eliminate waste products; 70 per cent of the body's waste products are eliminated through exhalation.
- Assisting the pumping of fluids about the body by the lymphatic pump and the cardiovascular pump. The lymphatic pump is essential for maintaining the health of our immune system – for people with asthma the healthier the immune system the better.
- Developing the 'relaxation response'. The sensation of breathlessness and restricted breathing easily creates frightening feelings of anxiety and panic. While this is entirely understandable, it's very important to know how to release muscle tension during asthma episodes. This helps reduce nervous as well as physical tension and 'turn down the volume' of the attack.

I developed asthma in my teens. At that time, my Ventolin and I were best buddies. The sheer fact of leaving my Ventolin inhaler behind would cause an episode to occur. I can remember going away without my inhaler and waking in the middle of the night needing it, the sensation of claustrophobia built quickly. All the time I was thinking: I'm stuck, all I need is that one puff. I needed my Ventolin.

Now I never use Ventolin, I am well medicated on my preventers. But I have also become aware of my breathing and I know what to do. Should I start to feel restriction in my chest, I stop and slow my breath down until I gain control. I haven't needed my Ventolin for the past few years, since I became aware of good breathing patterns and especially nose breathing. To be honest, if I didn't know this, I guarantee I would still be reaching for my Ventolin. **Duncan, 33**

Three main things that happen when we breathe

1. Breathing charges the blood with oxygen. Oxygen helps convert food into energy which powers the body and enables all cells to function; this is known as the metabolic process.

Breathing has an inverse relationship to energy; the rate, rhythm, depth and flow of our breaths will determine the quality and quantity of energy we receive.

If our breathing rate speeds up so does the amount of energy we use. For example, when we sprint our breathing is fast, explosive and peaked; the energy output is high. When we are tense and breathe into our upper chest the breath is faster, larger and sharper, and more energy is used. Large volumes are more demanding of muscular work, which also uses up more energy.

If the breathing rate slows down so does the energy we use. For example, in long-distance running the breath is easier, less peaked and well regulated; this gives endurance, as energy consumption is low over time.

When we are relaxed the breath is rhythmical, low and slow, and energy consumption is less.

As we say at Breathing Works, good breathing is like putting large amounts of money in the bank: at times we will withdraw and spend a lot of money – this occurs when our breathing speeds up in times of increased demand such as exertion, increased stress and demanding situations. But there is a problem if we spend too much, which is common in today's fast-paced society.

At the end of the day we must return to a balanced state, to allow recovery, normal functioning and optimum health. If we do not, ill health and chaos occur.

2. Breathing removes and maintains the levels of carbon dioxide required in the body. Carbon dioxide (CO_2) is the end result of the metabolic process. Although we all know how vital oxygen is, many people don't understand the importance of carbon dioxide. The carbon dioxide in our bodies regulates our breathing and our nervous system – the 'autonomic nervous system' which controls all our organs.

3. Breathing regulates the body's pH, i.e. the acid-alkaline balance. The pH in our body is no different from the pH in a swimming pool or in products such as shampoo or soap, in that they must all have a certain level of pH or they can be potentially harmful. The pH level in our bodies maintains our internal homeostasis, that is, the internal balance within our body. The pH level must stay the same; if this alters, a number of bodily changes occurs to try to regain the balance.

All three functions described above are essential for health, energy, vitality and wellbeing.

This places breathing as the overseer of everything that happens in our body: in short, if breathing is not right it is difficult for any bodily function to work properly.

CHAPTER 2

When good breathing goes bad

A crucial aspect of learning to live with asthma which is often ignored is the recognition of co-existing breathing pattern disorders. Muscles, such as the upper chest groups – supposed to be used in short bursts – are being asked to overwork 24 hours a day. These muscles use a lot of fuel. The lower chest muscles and diaphragm, built for endurance and minimum fuel consumption, weaken and find it harder to work as they were designed to.

Not only do the muscles themselves lose strength, but the messages from the brain – motor nerve pathways – also get diverted and send most of the instructions to the upper chest muscles instead of to the diaphragm. The natural lower chest breathing pattern has been overruled.

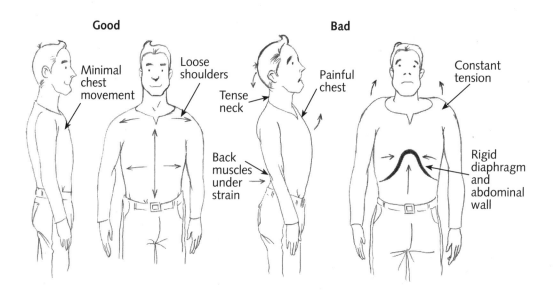

Good

Minimal chest movement
Loose shoulders
Tense neck
Back muscles under strain

Bad

Painful chest
Constant tension
Rigid diaphragm and abdominal wall

Mechanical problems

Disrupted breathing patterns mean that not only the breathing muscles are working at a terrible disadvantage, but also neck and shoulder muscles pull on supporting structures such as the spine, collarbones and base of the skull. Permanent changes in the way these muscles work mean disturbed breathing patterns become permanent too. This double-whammy can be both exhausting and painful, and in the long run, damaging. Muscle and ligament imbalances associated with asthma are commonly ignored. Upper chest tension leads to aches and pains. Joints and tendons are unable to work properly and are often stretched and strained, leading to damage and ongoing discomfort.

So if you continue with these faulty breathing patterns you're in danger of not only experiencing aches and pains but also triggering asthma symptoms – simply from the way you are breathing. The muscles used to continue these patterns need debriefing.

From early childhood the message is reinforced that what we breathe in – oxygen – is the most important thing. While this is true, it's only half true because what we breathe out – carbon dioxide – is of equal importance. Far from being just a waste gas at the end of the respiratory cycle, its presence – in balance with oxygen – is vital to our health.

Another childhood message that wends its way through to adult life is that of tightening the abdominal wall. ('Stand up straight, hold your stomach in!') The current gym culture perpetuates this. The very muscle that needs to work effectively and remain toned and elastic – the diaphragm – is forgotten.

Disturbed body chemistry

An extremely common breathing pattern disorder – fuelled by poorly tuned breathing muscles – is chronic hyperventilation. This means moving more air through the chest than the body can deal with while at rest. Too much carbon dioxide is huffed out, upsetting chemical balances in the body. People with asthma are sitting ducks for this sort of breathing pattern disorder.

The typical breathing pattern that brings this about is upper chest-breathing, and to add insult to injury, it is often partnered by habitual mouth-breathing. Raised shoulders, a hyperinflated upper chest and a slack jaw is the typical look (see picture below).

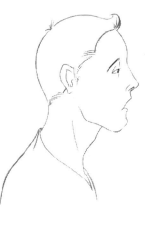 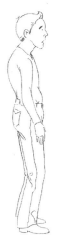

Mouth-breathing dries the airways   Slouching restricts the diaphragm

Most people, when they think of hyperventilation, think of acute episodes. These are very easy to spot. Breathing is visibly faster and louder than normal and the unpleasant or frightening symptoms caused by a sudden drop in CO_2 levels – racing heart or feeling faint, for instance – understandably lead to tension, anxiety or panicky feelings.

But chronic hyperventilation is more difficult to detect. People who have been habitually over-breathing for weeks, months or even years have reset the CO_2 monitor in their brains so the body accepts lower and fluctuating levels as normal. That's why so many chronic over-breathers complain of having 'good days and bad days' – and can never be sure what's happening, what triggered the feelings of unwellness, or why. Self-reliance takes a nose-dive.

When we over-breathe at rest or during normal low-level activity the following things can happen:

- Upper chest and/or mouth-breathing flushes out too much carbon dioxide from the body via the lungs.
- Mast cells, rather like watchdogs lying in the tissues supporting the airways, give warning signals to the airways activating higher histamine levels in the blood and triggering broncho-constriction (tight pipes) and

swelling of the linings of the airways. This is the lungs' attempt to keep foreign invaders from entering the airways.

- As the airways tighten in response to lower blood CO_2 levels, so do the arteries supplying other muscles, tissues and organs – including the brain. In fact, blood flow to the brain may be reduced by as much as 50 per cent during a bout of over-breathing. This often leads to feelings of suffocation and panic. It's hard to think clearly when this happens.

- Normal acid/alkaline balances (pH) in the body become altered. Over-breathing pushes CO_2 levels to lower than normal, which tends to make the body tissues more alkaline. Tingling and light-headedness may be the first signs of this. But continued or chronic over-breathing becomes more complex as the body tries to adjust long-term to this state of affairs. The kidneys are called in to excrete bicarbonate (alkaline), helping retain normal body acid. The drive to breathe faster becomes habitual to maintain a normal pH (the body takes great pains to preserve this). CO_2 levels remain lowered and the respiratory centre in the brain learns to accept this. The rest of the body is not quite so accepting. It suffers.

- Low CO_2 also stimulates lactic acid build-up in body cells as they attempt to balance their pH and metabolism is affected. Muscles ache, particularly the overused upper chest. These muscles are greedy for oxygen, stealing it away from lower back and leg muscles which may be extra painful during exercise. Chronic tiredness and exhaustion follow.

The autonomic nervous system

The autonomic nervous system (ANS) which looks after the automatic functions of the body – such as heart rate, digestion and blood pressure – is affected too.

The ANS is divided into two:

the **sympathetic** branch which speeds us up,

and the **parasympathetic** branch which calms us down.

Low CO_2 levels provoke the sympathetic nervous system more than the parasympathetic, putting the body – and mind – on 'red alert'. This includes the airways, which may tighten and cause asthma.

In ancient times, when our ancestors lived in caves, fear (sympathetic nervous system stimulation) prepared prehistoric tribes for 'fright, flight, fight'. Adrenalin poured into the bloodstream. Pupils dilated, heart and breathing rates sped up, airways relaxed to prepare the body for immediate danger and action.

The modern version of this ancient response is prolonged exposure to stressful events such as noisy traffic, school, the workplace, or stressful family or social interactions. The body starts to 'contract' – muscles tighten, breathing and heart rates increase, blood vessels and airways tighten.

Prolonged sympathetic stimulation, along with low CO_2 levels caused by over-breathing, may double up to trigger asthma symptoms.

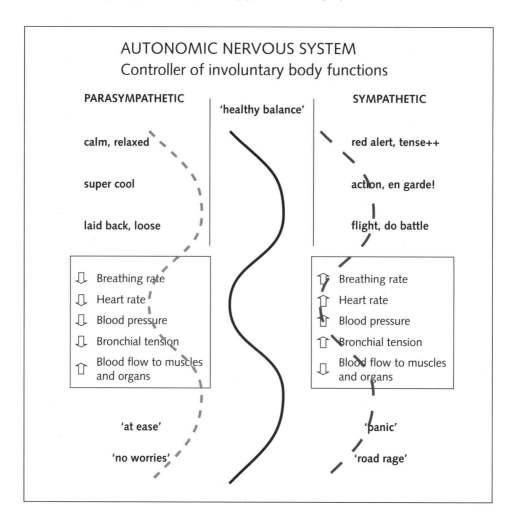

Someone in the throes of a severe asthma attack usually switches unconsciously between upper chest and abdominal breathing, as either group of muscles tires. This is entirely normal. During a sudden severe or prolonged episode, carbon dioxide levels may begin to rise as oxygen levels fall because of broncho-constriction and extra mucus production preventing sufficient air from entering the lungs. The brain has a switch that speeds up breathing when CO_2 rises above a healthy level. (It needs to speed up to dispose of the excess CO_2.) This is not the time to practise perfect breathing! Assuming a Rest Position (see page 38) to help the breathing muscles work as efficiently and effectively as they can while waiting for asthma medications to work – as well as encourage relaxation – is the best option at this time.

Making sure your breathing stays good

If you have been newly diagnosed with asthma you've probably been armed with Medication Plans, Action Plans to monitor symptoms, and new user-friendly inhalers to help you breathe freely again. Asthma education is essential to understand what is going on in your airways and the reason behind the choices of medication prescribed. Of equal importance is to check that your breathing rates and patterns return to 'normal' when you get relief from your asthma symptoms. Musculo-skeletal changes may lock you into bad breathing patterns, with prolonged sympathetic nervous system dominance making fertile ground for asthma to flourish.

If you've had asthma for any length of time, chances are you may be a long-time 'bad breather'. It's not always possible to manage breathing retraining on your own. In fact, it can be downright difficult. Breathing lessons may be an essential part of Asthma education for you.

CHAPTER 3

It's right under your nose

As I watched my baby breathe I realised he could only use his nose. Even when he had a cold he would struggle to get air through his nostrils and only when it became too difficult almost to suffocation point would he open his mouth to cry, like a pressure valve being released, stealing a mouth-breath to fill his lungs. He did not know how to mouth-breathe; mouth-breathing is a learnt response triggered by emergency situations.

Tania, mother of Oliver, 6 months

How does the nose affect my asthma?

Nasal problems are extremely common in the general population – chronic rhinitis, allergic rhinitis (hay fever), sinusitis and post-nasal drip are rife amongst people with asthma.

There is a nerve reflex connecting the nose to our airways which acts like a trip-wire, so that when the nose is affected by an allergen or congestion this can also trigger off broncho-constriction.

We know that there are nerve connections between the bronchi and the sinuses. There is a condition called sinobronchial syndrome in which if the sinuses are congested they will cause broncho-spasm in the bronchial airways. The treatment involves clearance of the sinuses.

Nose versus mouth

Breathing through the nose creates 50 per cent more airflow resistance than breathing through the mouth. No wonder many of us take the easy option and use our mouths! This is particularly true during exercise and stressful situations.

Air is streamlined through the nose, allowing lesser amounts compared to mouth-breathing. Most of us think more is better, but as we have seen in Chapter 2 this is not the case. Too much air or over-breathing can lead to cases of chronic hyperventilation. With nose-breathing, air enters the body in a more controlled flow, making acute hyperventilation virtually impossible.

If your nose is blocked you will start mouth-breathing. The problem with mouth-breathing is that it allows cool, dry, unfiltered air into the lungs – a little like rubbing sandpaper over your skin. This causes irritation which can lead to asthma.

The mouth is there for emergencies. We know that when we mouth-breathe quickly this has a direct link to our autonomic nervous system, triggering the sympathetic 'flight and fight' branch that readies us for emergencies.

If you don't use it you lose it: the more we use our nose the better it works.

Why is the nose so important?

The nose is our air-conditioning system that prepares and cleanses the air for delivery into the body. Its three main functions are to moisten the air, to warm the air, and to filter out impurities that are carried in the air.

The nose has a protective mucosal lining inside the nasal cavity, similar to the lining in the passages of the airways. Foreign particles stick to this lining and are then blown and sneezed out. Sneezing can throw things out of our nose at amazing speeds: air can leave our nose at a speed of 160 km/h.

The nose produces a gas called nitric oxide (NO). Recent research on the nose suggests that this gas may have a role in:

- sterilising incoming air,
- maintaining mucociliary clearance; this prevents mucus from pooling and becoming infected,
- acting as a messenger for blood flow and oxygen uptake, thus ensuring good oxygenation to the body and
- the nose is also believed to be an arterial and bronchial vasodilator, helping to keep the airways open – which for asthma we know is a vital and key function.

Other functions of the nose

- It links smell to experiences and emotion; for example, the smell of a strong brew of coffee or the smell of perfume reminding us of certain places or people.
- It directs the airflow, which determines our physical endurance; e.g. in racehorses it used to be the practice to clip the inside of their nostrils to 'help' them run faster.
- It creates a pressure difference between the nose and lungs, which allows efficient gas exchange to occur; i.e. it ensures oxygen is transported to the body. Nose-breathing has a far higher pressure gradient than mouth-breathing, allowing energy-efficient breathing to occur.

The structures

The structures that make up the nose are quite complex, and to understand them you almost require an engineering degree.

The nose is divided into two narrow cavities by the septum, made of bone and cartilage; this allows each side to function as a separate unit. The nostrils at the opening of these cavities are lined with fine hairs which filter out dust and bacteria. Deeper in the cavity lie the turbinates.

The turbinates are characterised by three ridges of bone which regulate the airflow in the nostrils. The turbinate is lined with a mucosal lining which has a rich blood supply; this performs the function of warming and humidifying the air, ready for its inhalation into the body. The lining produces mucus daily, which clears dust, grime and microbes such as viruses and bacteria out of the air; it has been estimated that we inhale 20 billion particles of foreign matter a day. Hence the importance of keeping mucus flowing, as if it pools for too long it can rapidly become infected.

The cilia are hair-like structures that are responsible for clearing the mucus away; they work like oars moving at 16 strokes a second. If the mucus becomes too thick or thin they become ineffective.

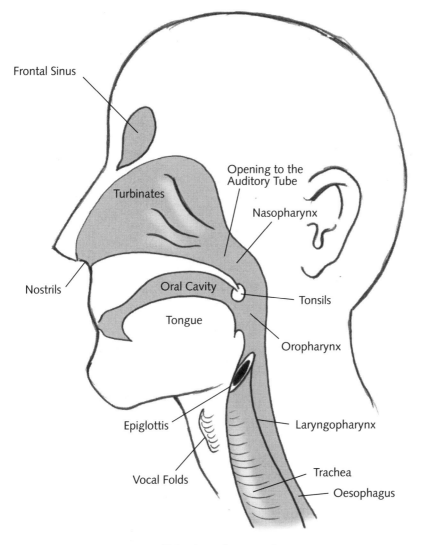

Frontal Sinus

Opening to the
Auditory Tube

Turbinates

Nasopharynx

Nostrils

Oral Cavity

Tonsils

Tongue

Oropharynx

Epiglottis

Laryngopharynx

Vocal Folds

Trachea

Oesophagus

Side view of upper airways

The sinuses are air-filled cavities surrounding the main nasal cavity. They assist
in the warming and filtering of air, and also to make sound – working as echo
chambers.

Small passages from the sinuses lead into the nasal cavity, allowing for the
removal of mucus; it is easy for these passages to become blocked, which
creates pressure, and as a result sinus headaches occur.

Mucus is cleared via nasal blowing, or swallowing.

Specific conditions

Sinusitis

Many people who have asthma have sinusitis as well. Sinusitis is caused by a bacterial infection in the sinuses. Acute sinusitis often comes on after a cold or infection and lasts a few weeks; chronic sinusitis usually starts with nasal inflammation, which leads to blocked cavities, which in turn become infected with bacteria. This can become a vicious cycle that is difficult to treat.

Sinus pain comes from pressure on the membranes in the cavities. The worst pain occurs when a vacuum is formed, for example when flying at high altitudes.

For treatment of sinusitis see your GP who will prescribe the right medication. There are also things you can do for yourself:

- Daily nasal washes (see page 30)
- Tractions to the sinuses to assist the movement of the mucus (see picture on page 31)
- If your sinuses are infected use the steam inhalation technique and the drainage positions for effective sputum clearance (see pages 31, 32)
- Hot compresses to the sinuses to assist cilia movement
- Postural exercises to relieve sinus pressures (see Chapter 10)

The aim of the treatment is to help restore the movement of the cilia in the nose and sinuses.

Hay fever: allergic rhinitis

Hay fever is an allergy to airborne pollen; hence its other name, allergic rhinitis. It is generally characterised by sneezing, and/or a runny nose, itchy, watery eyes, and a blocked nose, generally making one feel miserable – certainly making it difficult for kissing!

If you suffer from hay fever it is a good idea to address this, as often your asthma will improve as a result.

For treatment of hay fever, see your GP for the proper nasal spray, antihistamines and allergy tests. Things you can do for yourself are:

- Nasal washes (see page 30)
- Traction (see picture on page 31)
- Good breathing patterns (see Chapter 7)
- Postural stretching (see Chapter 10)

Post-nasal drip

This refers to the sensation of thick phlegm in the throat. It often occurs as a result of the nasal ciliary system slowing down. The treatment for this is to restore healthy function to the cilia mucosal system by using nasal washes.

Nasal polyps

These are non-cancerous tumours that grow in the mucous membranes of the nose. They occur commonly in people with allergies.

Early-morning sneezing

This is often caused by the nose trying to get rid of particles that have accumulated overnight. If the cilia are working well this should not occur; however, cilia do not work as well in cool situations. The other reason this can occur is if allergies are severe, meaning that our body's thermostat does not work as well.

Warming up prior to getting out of bed speeds up the cilia and sneezing is avoided. There's nothing like a good hot cup of tea!

Children and ear infections

Often children who have recurring ear problems are chronic mouth-breathers. With the altered mouth-breathing pattern the lymphatic flow is disturbed and becomes stagnant in the region of the head and neck; fluid pools in the middle ear, providing an ideal environment for bacteria and hence infection. So it is a good idea, if your child is predisposed to ear infections, to check their breathing pattern.

Mothers in Eastern countries train their babies to nose-breathe by tipping their heads forward when they sleep; this closes the lips and makes nostril-breathing unavoidable.

Mouth-breathers

Some of us have been mouth-breathers for years. There are many reasons for this to occur, and as with all breathing pattern disorders, once the pattern becomes 'hard-wired' we think it is normal.

Steps towards healthy nose-breathing

It takes time to recondition the body to use the nose – anything from three weeks to months. Start with the steps on page 54 and then follow on with the Breathing Works nasal hygiene regime (see below).

Clearance methods

Salt water is a natural wash for the linings of the nasal cavity: the cavity is accustomed to such a composition as tears, which are salty and drain into the nose along the sinuses. It is well known that people who regularly swim in the sea have excellent nasal health.

> ### Nasal wash recipe
> This recipe for a nasal wash is an easy, cheap and effective remedy. Salt is a preservative so it won't 'go off'.
>
> Dissolve $1/2$ teaspoon of rock or sea salt (this helps to reduce nasal sogginess) and $1/2$ teaspoon of bicarbonate of soda (this acts like Teflon so nothing can stick) in 500 mls of boiled water. Wait for this to cool, then fill a sterilised, recycled nasal spray bottle or bulb syringe with the solution and discard the rest.
>
> Spray each nostril morning and evening for two to three days: spray until you feel it hit the back of your throat, with the spray bottle almost horizontal for maximum saturation. Aim the nozzle towards the outside corner of the eye on the same side as the nostril being sprayed. Sniff gently, hoick and spit. Spray as required.

The 'snuffle' method: Wash and dry your hands before pouring some of the above solution into the palm of your hand; closing one nostril, snuffle the saline into your nose. Move the jaw a couple of times to allow movement of the fluid along the sinuses and blow out. If the water goes into the upper sinuses you may experience an unpleasant, stinging sensation. This will not harm you, so please don't let it deter you – we cannot emphasise enough the importance of healthy clear passages.

Repeat and do two palmfuls up the other nostril. This method suits those who don't like using or are fed up with gadgets.

If you have a nasal infection rinse with the nasal wash twice a day, morning and night, until the infection improves. The rinse can also be used as a mouth gargle when you have a sore throat or generally to cleanse the mouth and throat.

Steam inhalation

Use this when you have a nasal infection, twice a day for two weeks.

Boil water in a pot, or the jug, allow to cool for a few minutes, then lean over the water with a towel draped over your head; inhale the steam. You can add friar's balsam or Vicks Vaporub for added punch.

Physical methods

Traction

Pressure applied to the small bones that make up the sinuses is an ideal way to relieve pressure. Looking at the picture shown, place your fingers on the spots marked X. Then press and pull gently in the arrowed direction. Hold for 10 seconds, repeat three times.

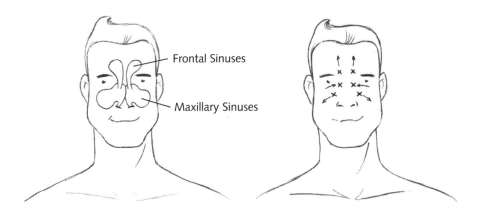

Frontal Sinuses

Maxillary Sinuses

Acupressure

1. Pressure is placed on the lower surface of your clavicle (collarbone) where it joins the sternum (breastbone). Press in this region; holding gently, place pressure upwards as if to lift the collarbone – hold for the count of 10. This does several things:

- It helps decrease nasal obstruction.
- It also assists lymphatic movement which helps removal of waste products and maintenance of a healthy immune system.

2. Pressure is placed on the first rib. Hold this area and pull downwards as you breathe out; this assists with the release of air from the nose. It is a brilliant exercise if you are prone to breath-holding.

Head positioning for nasal drainage

While lying down turn your head 45 degrees on your pillow and stay in this position for up to 10 minutes; then change sides. This allows drainage of the maxillary sinuses.

Postural stretches

For adequate nasal functioning it is important that there is mobility in the region of the mid back. For mechanically efficient breathing, see stretches on pages 85–86.

Nasal medication

If your doctor prescribes nasal medication, ensure you know exactly what it is for, why you are taking it and how to use it. Ask about and be prepared for any side-effects.

Nasal medications fall into two groups:

- Relievers: These cause shrinkage of the nasal linings. They should not be used continuously, as overuse can make the nose clog up even more.
- Preventers: These have long-term, anti-inflammatory and anti-allergic benefits. They are usually local steroids (sprayed up the nose), which coat the lining of the nose with minimal effect on the rest of the body. Commitment to regular use is essential to get the full benefit.

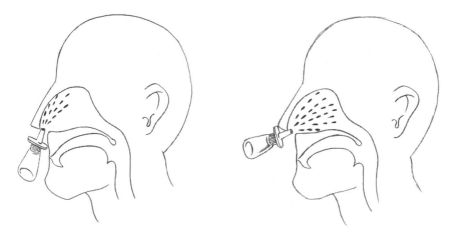

Aim the nozzle towards the outside corner of the eye of the same side
as the nostril being sprayed.

Nose-blowing

If this is too violent it can cause sinus and ear problems. The best way to blow
your nose and prevent damage to the tubes that connect with the inner ear is
to block off one nostril while clearing the other gently. This is very important,
especially for young children.

So the nose is it: the first port of call for good breathing and a prerequisite
for ALL health.

CHAPTER 4

The vital pump

I can't describe the feeling, when I actually felt my stomach wall relax and I breathed low in my chest. It felt so foreign, but at the same time familiar! And the feeling of letting go and relaxing was utterly wonderful. **Susan, 61**

The diaphragm has been called the vital pump. This fabulous, unheralded muscle helps the body in so many ways, yet rarely receives the acclaim it deserves. While the heart grabs all the attention as the primary pump propelling blood around the body, the diaphragm quietly provides the oxygen needed to nourish and fuel us. It also helps the lungs to exhale the by-product of energy consumption – carbon dioxide.

As well as being the main pump providing oxygen via the lungs to all the body's tissues and organs, the diaphragm helps in many other areas. Described as 'the muscular equivalent of an umbilical cord', the diaphragm takes over at birth, linking us to the outside world and keeping us alive.

Examine this illustration and look at the attachments and boundaries of this amazing muscle. We can neither see it nor feel it and yet it pumps – mostly without complaint – all our lives, round the clock, 15–23,000 times a day (and many more if you are a chronic over-breather).

Lower tip of the sternum

Rib margins

Spinal attachment

Two common complaints
- **Hiccoughs.** These occur when our diaphragms react to insults such as eating or drinking too fast. The stomach becomes over-stretched and presses up onto the diaphragm; this irritates it, either directly or via the nerves sending signals to it. Spasms or uncontrollable contractions across the diaphragm draw air in quickly and unexpectedly, causing the epiglottis in the throat to snap shut.
- **'Stitch'** is thought to be caused by the diaphragm not receiving enough oxygen to work effectively. It is usually felt during vigorous exercise: one theory is that abdominal organs hitting up against the muscular fibres of the diaphragm cause it to spasm. Another theory is lack of blood supply to the diaphragm when blood may have been diverted to the digestive tract if exercise is taken too soon after food.

How the diaphragm works

Imagine your chest is like a birdcage, the bony ribs supporting and protecting the delicate spongy lungs within. These fill with air with that first gasp at birth and remain inflated throughout life. The lungs sit on the dome of the diaphragm which separates them from the gut. As the diaphragm flattens and descends during inspiration, the lung tissue is gently expanded to allow fresh oxygen-rich air to flow in. Your stomach wall relaxes and expands to allow this. As you breathe out, the elastic recoil of both your stomach wall and the rising diaphragm effortlessly expels used carbon dioxide-rich air. There is minimal use of energy.

Compare this to raising up and contracting back your ribcage with upper chest-breathing; here there is *maximum* use of energy. The diaphragm is unable to work at its energy-efficient best when upper chest-breathing becomes the norm. This is a very common pattern in people with asthma. It's sometimes referred to as 'reverse breathing'.

Although it is entirely normal to use your upper chest muscles during heavy exercise, excitement, or during a bout of asthma, it's very important to debrief them, switch them off, and restore normal nose/belly breathing again. Breathing retraining helps to do this.

One way you can get a hint of the work your diaphragm does is by means of the 'sniff test'. Place your hands on your stomach just below the V of your ribs. Take a quick sniff in through your nose and feel the quick outward movement of your stomach wall, as the diaphragm contracts and flattens. Chronic upper-chest breathers tend to do the opposite so this test is useful in identifying a chronic upper-chest breather. Try it yourself. If you 'sniffed' into your upper chest you may need a breathing lesson.

An unexpected bonus from my breathing retraining was the improvement of my reflux problems. I was able to stop taking my 'heartburn' pills and my digestion really improved. **Bill, 42**

Other important functions of the diaphragm

Digestion

The food we eat travels down the oesophagus, through the chest, and via a valve, crosses the diaphragm into the stomach. This valve prevents food regurgitating back up the oesphagus. The musculature of the diaphragm surrounding the valve helps maintain its strength and efficiency. A diaphragm that is not working properly is not going to be of any help to the oesophageal valve in preventing uncomfortable disorders such as 'heartburn', indigestion and gastric reflux. Remember the diaphragm muscle is like any other skeletal muscle – it will weaken with disuse. A strong working diaphragm helps reduce these problems.

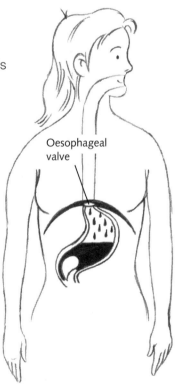

Oesophageal valve

Another valuable digestive function of the diaphragm is its gentle massaging of the stomach and gut, as it moves up and down with normal breathing. People with Irritable Bowel Syndrome are invariably found to be 'bad breathers'.

This same gentle pumping action helps with lymph flow, through the pelvis, stomach and chest. Our auto-immune system relies on efficient lymph circulation through the various channels and clusters of lymph nodes to maintain health.

The great blood vessels from the lower part of the body traverse the diaphragm too, through valves which also need strong support. Blood returning to the heart from the legs has to overcome gravity. The pumping action of the diaphragm also helps the heart in this way.

Speaking

People with asthma – particularly if they are feeling slightly wheezy – are notorious for upper chest-breathing while speaking. Gasping in large draughts of air with upper chest bracing, their voices sound strained and sometimes husky. They are also at risk of forcing out too much CO_2, leading to symptoms such as light-headedness or 'stage fright'. A strong diaphragm helps produce a confident flowing pattern of speech, essential for people who rely on their voices – such as actors, telephonists, lawyers, teachers or broadcasters.

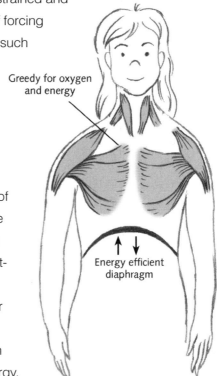

Greedy for oxygen and energy

Energy efficient diaphragm

If none of the above considerations of the diaphragm motivates you to become an abdominal breather, consider this. At rest and during mild activity, upper chest-breathing gobbles up between **10–30 per cent** of your available energy. Upper chest muscles are **greedy**. Using the diaphragm reduces this cost to between **2–4 per cent**. Don't waste precious energy. Turbocharge your diaphragm!

During an asthma attack take up a Rest Position to reduce shoulder tension and help the diaphragm work its best for you. See below.

Rest Positions

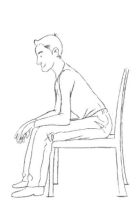
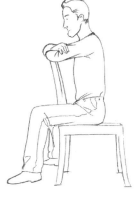
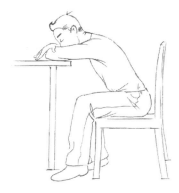
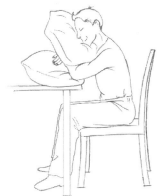
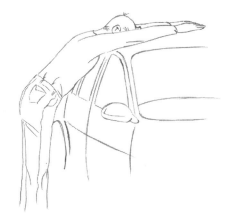

CHAPTER 5

Body works

It all started after a six-week period of increased pressure at work. I couldn't get a decent breath, my whole body ached, I had pains, especially in my arms, forearms and my hands, and I felt giddy and sick. I even got to the point of dropping things. All this time I thought the only thing I could do was to keep increasing my reliever – I would use it sometimes eight or nine times a day. Understandably, by the time I saw my GP he couldn't believe the state I had got into.

After improving my awareness and re-education of my breathing pattern my symptoms have improved – I only take my reliever prior to exercise now, and that is more as a precautionary measure. I have specific stretching exercises to do as I am at a computer all day. I can now see how the combination of poor breathing patterns developed over a lifetime of asthma, increased pressure and the type of work I do led to the spiralling of my problem. All I can say is thank goodness for low, slow nose-breathing. **Rebecca, 30**

You have been introduced to the main breathing muscles in Chapter 1 and the diaphragm in Chapter 4. To understand fully the importance of correct patterns of energy-efficient breathing we will look at the structures in more detail.

The fasciae

The body has tissues, called fasciae, that surround the muscle layers. The fasciae envelop the soft tissues, rather like clingfilm. The fasciae extend from the top of your head to the tips of your toes. There are, however, areas where they change like the seams in a dress. There is a dominant fascia running from the base of the head to the top of the diaphragm, encasing the heart on its journey. Whenever we breathe it is the movement of this fascia that micro-massages the heart and all the structures involved with it.

In fact, it has been said that all parts of the body are in direct or indirect relationship to the diaphragm.

The muscles

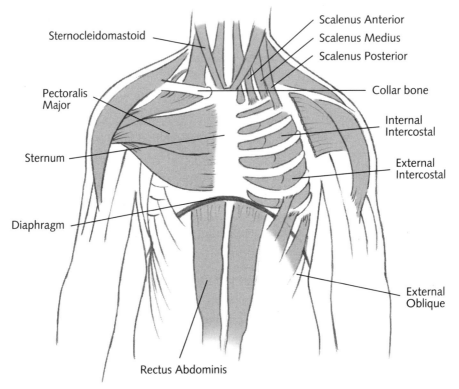

Sternocleidomastoid

Scalenus Anterior
Scalenus Medius
Scalenus Posterior

Pectoralis Major

Collar bone

Internal Intercostal

Sternum

External Intercostal

Diaphragm

External Oblique

Rectus Abdominis

Inhalation

Main breathing muscles:

The diaphragm see chapter 4

Scalenes

These lift and help to expand the ribcage during inspiration. They are active with each breath, increasing in use with high demands.

Intercostal muscles

The external intercostal muscles sit between the ribs. They work to close and expand the ribcage.

Muscles that assist in breathing: sternocleidomastoids

These muscles connect the head to your shoulder girdle. Their main function is to stabilise the head, but they can be used for breathing, especially in situations of exertion or stress. Imagine an asthma attack or a time when you have been short of breath. Think about how you have been breathing – imagine looking at yourself in the mirror. What do you think your breathing pattern looks like? See your chest heaving. The muscles doing a lot of the work of breathing are the sternocleidomastoids and the scalenes; it is easy for these muscles to become overused and overworked. The body follows the head, so if there is any tightness or overuse in these muscles we end up with a very poor posture (see page 65).

Other chest muscles called the pectoralis muscles work on breathing when our arms are elevated.

Exhalation

The trunk and abdominal muscles assist in forced exhalation; they also play a large role in pressure, volume control and stability.

The abdominals are accessory expiratory muscles of great strength: without these muscles our bellies would bulge outward from the pressure of the abdominal contents. The action of the abdominal muscles is essential for the efficiency of the diaphragm; they work in opposition to, and in conjunction with, the diaphragm in breathing. The combined movement of the diaphragm and the abdomen is like a 'push-me-pull-you': when the diaphragm contracts the abdomen relaxes, and when the diaphragm retracts, retraction of the abdominals occurs.

The diaphragm would be less effective in the absence of abdominal muscles.

Maintaining the balance

Stability is created when there is a balance between the muscles of the pelvic floor, trunk, abdomen and diaphragm. This stability is vital for correct posture, movement and body propulsion. Stability maintains the ideal posture and keeps the body neutral in all movements (Chapter 8 describes 'the body neutral' in more detail).

The deep abdominal muscles work to maintain stability anteriorly; if these are not strong the central tendon of the diaphragm would not be stabilised, allowing the diaphragm to elevate the lower ribs.

We have seen that when we breathe in, the diaphragm pushes down, increasing the vertical diameter of the thorax. This movement is opposed by our abdominal contents, the stomach and pelvic floor muscles. These muscles need to be firm to maintain pressure: you can imagine what happens if we have weak muscles; there is no resistance and we would end up with inefficient breathing and the beginning of a bad pattern.

Imagine a cardboard box: when we place pressure on the top, if all sides are firm the pressure will be absorbed, but if any side is weak the box will collapse – our posture and breathing work in a similar way.

If breathing changes are maintained for long periods, the ratio of muscular use also alters, and the neck and shoulder muscles, which are our emergency muscles, start to work more frequently. In time they often become the main breathing muscles instead of the diaphragm. This leads to a reversed pattern of breathing which has many adverse effects, such as inefficient posture.

Decreased diaphragm movement

The loss of diaphragm movement sets up a sequence of events leading to inefficient breathing patterns.

Loss of the pumping action of the diaphragm

This results in the loss of micro-massaging to all internal organs. Weakness of the muscles surrounding the oesophageal valve results in reflux and gut problems, and also in the loss of fluid being pumped to the cardiovascular and lymphatic systems. This results in venous pooling in the legs and an inefficient lymphatic system, which in turn creates an inefficient immune system.

Loss of lower rib movement

This leads to the loss of micro-massaging to the spinal column, resulting in rigidity, stiffness and ultimately pain.

Pelvic floor weakness

This results in bladder problems and weak spinal stabilising muscles.

Abdominal and spinal muscles end up imbalanced

This leads to postural dysfunction and pain.

Fascial restriction – from the neck to the diaphragm

This leads to poor posture, immobility of structures and ligaments, and the loss of micro-massaging to the heart.

Rib movement loss

Second rib loss of movement causes decreased lymphatic and blood circulation. Loss of lymphatic movement has an effect on our immune system.

Rigid cervical (neck) and thoracic (mid back) vertebrae

This results in pain and loss of movement. The nervous system is also affected, as the spine houses and protects the spinal cord and nerve roots.

Accessory muscle overuse

Accessory muscle overuse leads to a build-up of lactic acid in the overused muscle, resulting in pain and discomfort. A reduced blood supply to the arms and legs due to a reduction in CO_2 levels in the blood from over-breathing will further add to the discomfort and pain. These muscles become tight and stiff and as a result postural changes occur, causing dysfunction in the whole body. If this continues, problems can become chronic. This is commonly seen in disorders such as Occupational Overuse Syndrome.

Another factor of the tight musculature is impingement of vital structures such as the brachial artery and brachial nerve plexus (see picture). If the brachial plexuses between the scalene muscles become overused and tight, the nerve plexus is affected, causing discomfort and problems in the arms.

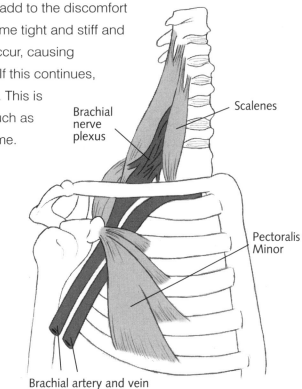

Brachial nerve plexus

Scalenes

Pectoralis Minor

Brachial artery and vein

Recent studies in Australia show the significance of good diaphragm breathing for lower back health. Where the diaphragm inserts into the spine (see page 34), with each energy-efficient breath there is a massaging effect, creating a good blood supply and good spinal health – yet again, poor patterns can lead to chronic lower back problems.

If the above malfunctions continue, other compounding problems can occur – headaches, backache, sinus problems, jaw problems, achy body, sleep deprivation... This is just some of what can happen – and of course we expect the worsening of asthma symptoms and reduced control of your asthma.

Whew! What can you do?

A good start is to achieve energy-efficient breathing patterns. Follow the Breathing Works method, described in Chapter 7, followed by good posture (Chapter 8) and maintain mobility (Chapter 10). Good luck!

CHAPTER 6

Coughing

No one needs to be taught to cough. It's the body's strongest physiological reflex, designed to keep airways clear. It's normal to have about half a teacup of clear mucus spread over the surfaces of all the airways, large and small, at any one time. Swept round by the action of tiny hairs, or cilia, it helps remove inhaled dust or irritants.

During asthma episodes these little hairs or sweepers can become overwhelmed as mucus builds up. Coughing is therefore a very common symptom of asthma, when soggy airways need to be cleared. Unfortunately it can also cause broncho- constriction or 'tight pipes'. The more the airways are obstructed, the weaker the cough.

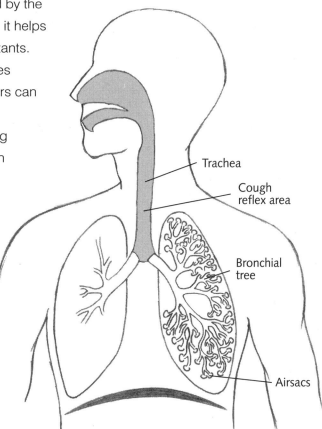

Trachea

Cough reflex area

Bronchial tree

Airsacs

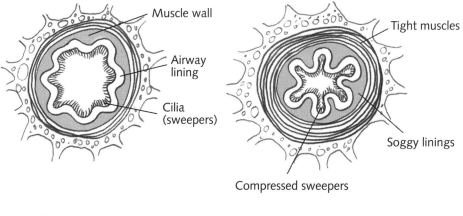

Muscle wall

Airway lining

Cilia (sweepers)

Tight muscles

Soggy linings

Compressed sweepers

Normal airways
cross-section

In asthma
cross-section

Fortunately coughing can also be controlled at will, and learning 'cough control' methods helps reduce the panicky feelings that accompany chest tightness. Prescribed bronchodilator drugs may be used to help relax the airways, while the gentle breathing and cough manoeuvres clear the mucus.

The ACBT

Since the early 1990s the Active Cycle of Breathing Technique (ACBT) has superseded an older Forced Expiratory Technique (FET) as a physiotherapeutic chest clearance method. The former has the advantage of relaxed abdominal breathing as part of the cycle and is a much gentler way of 'milking' the lower airways of mucus build-up. The latter was found to be too vigorous for people with asthma and ran the risk of making symptoms worse. So if you're still practising the old way – update now.

DEEP versus BIG breaths

Most people when asked to take a deep breath immediately breathe in through their mouth or noisily through their nose, expanding their upper chests and in some cases sucking in their stomachs! That's a BIG breath – fine for blowing out birthday candles. DEEP breathing is nose, low chest, abdominal breaths where your stomach *gently* expands as you breathe in, and relaxes as you breathe out. There is *minimal* upper chest involvement. Try them both and note the difference.

The ACBT alternates between:

- Relaxed abdominal nose (deep) breathing – five to six breaths.
- Two full (big) breaths, filling the chest gently via the nose, and letting go so the air *whooshes* quietly out of your chest through your mouth. There is no breath-holding, pushing or force used during these two full chest breaths.

Repeat this cycle three to four times.

Then try two huffs. This is done by breathing in only *halfway* before huffing out – (rather like huffing on a mirror before polishing it). You should feel your stomach wall tighten in, as you huff out.

If you can hear a rattle or feel any mucus, cough twice – no more – to bring it out. If it remains stuck, don't keep coughing; go through the whole cycle again and again until it becomes easier to cough up.

Repeat the cycle until the huff sounds dry.

Always finish with relaxed nose, belly breathing.

You can practise in lying, side-lying, sitting or standing postures. In short, anywhere, any time.

Analysing the cycle

You can appreciate that by using relaxed abdominal breathing and the diaphragm, the lower lobes of the lungs are going to be expanded.

The next step – the two full chest breaths – takes the airways by surprise and the sudden increased volumes help to shear mucus from the airways.

Repetition gets things moving. The huffs complete the cycle by gently propelling phlegm up to the cough reflex area. Coughing is then much more effective. Breathing becomes easier.

It is very important to do **all the phases of the cycle** – and always to finish with *relaxed*, *low*, *slow*, *nose*, *belly breathing*. It's a simple way of keeping ahead of mucus production and helping prevent chest infections.

Other options

There are various 'flutter' devices on the market that provide fine vibrations down the airways as you breathe out through the device. Shaped rather like a 'spacer', they are very easy to use and are particularly good if there is a lot of mucus, and your cough has become very weak or ineffectual. The gentle vibration shakes mucus loose and combined with abdominal breathing, helps clear the chest. We recommend the Acapella® positive expiratory pressure (PEP) device which has a detachable mouthpiece and optional mask; it can be used while sitting upright or lying down. It comes in adult and children's sizes. (See Useful Resources on page 110 for further information.)

Shake, rattle and roll

Keeping the obstructed airways free of mucus in the early stages of a chest infection is an often-forgotten **first line of defence**; using the ACBT and/or flutter device with gravity assistance by lying over pillows or cushions can be extremely effective.

Having someone tap your back ('tip and huff') is an added bonus, by gently vibrating the chest wall and helping loosen mucus build-up and relieve muscle tensions. Children especially enjoy this and as the ACBT is sometimes difficult to get children to perform, it may be another option if done carefully, with gentle relaxing massage as well. Kids often prefer the more active approach – and they appreciate the physical contact and attention, particularly if they have been frightened by their symptoms.

If you decide to 'tip and huff' – make sure you have an empty bladder and tissues to spit into. Flush them down the lavatory when you've finished coughing. *Don't leave them lying around and don't forget to wash your hands.*

'Coughing up'

Some find the whole notion of chest clearance disgusting and cannot/will not 'cough up'. Swallowing is perfectly normal. Younger children tend to do this; however, excessive mucus is better out than in. It's also an opportunity to quickly check to see what colour the phlegm might be. Pale cream or yellowy hues usually indicate allergic or inflammatory responses, while darker or greenish tones mean infection.

Whether to increase preventers or start a course of antibiotics can be decided on these observations. Doctors often like to send a 'sputum sample' for investigation, to make sure the right sort of antibiotic is chosen for the particular type of bug. This helps reduce the risk of having to take repeated courses if the first one fails to work.

Take care to complete each course of antibiotics, and contact your doctor immediately if you experience a bad reaction.

Irritable coughing

Sometimes coughing can be triggered by dry, irritable upper airways. It comes as no surprise that this often stems from *chronic mouth-breathing*. Sometimes it starts as a response to stress, and tightening of throat muscles. The continued high-velocity airflow via the mouth 'roughs up' the already irritated airway linings; the habit of constant throat clearing or coughing perpetuates the cycle.

Sometimes poor inhaler techniques mean medications hit the back of the throat, causing huskiness and irritation (see page 101).

Becoming a nose breather is top priority, and often this is enough to calm down an aggravated throat. But where a bad habit has taken hold, the following course of action may be necessary.

Dry cough patrol

To help break the cycle of unproductive cough – irritation – more coughing – drying of upper airways – more irritation – coughing – wheezing, learn to

- nose breathe
- abdominal breathe, low and slow, at low volumes
- take small sips of water *very frequently* – always have a glass of water or water-bottle with you *at all times* to keep your upper airways well sluiced
- suck small liquorice-based pastilles or other over-the-counter throat lozenges before telephoning/speaking for long periods.

Suppress the sometimes overwhelming desire to cough by:

- swallowing hard
- dropping/relaxing your shoulders
- concentrating on breathing out gently

Learning how to cough effectively reduces the risk of 'tight pipes' (broncho-spasm). Uncontrolled cough velocities may reach as high as 100 km/h. Common side-effects from tight or violent hacking coughs are headaches and painful neck, shoulder and chest muscles. It can be tough on your bladder too. Leaking during bouts of coughing may take you by surprise. Make sure you tighten these muscles before coughing.

Check your pelvic floor strength by trying, next time you empty your bladder, to stop the flow of urine about halfway through. *This applies to men as well as women.* If you can't, you'll need to tone up your pelvic floor muscles. Also, use the less explosive, airway-friendly and effective methods of cough control described above. Be kind to your airways.

If you have any difficulties, check with your physiotherapist.

CHAPTER 7

A recipe for good breathing patterns

I thought my doctor was nuts, suggesting I have breathing lessons.
I've been breathing all my life, haven't I? What else is there to
know? I grudgingly agreed and I must say, I learned a lot. It was
harder than I thought but the pay-off has been great. My puffer use
has gone way down. **Peter, 27**

The first ingredient is commitment. Regular practice is essential, *even as you
start to feel better*. It takes from six to eight weeks to change from faulty to
'normal' breathing patterns, providing practice is consistently regular.

Remember you were hard-wired at birth to nose/diaphragm-breathe. The
pattern is there, even if it is deeply buried beneath newer defective ones.
Some people may take longer than others to unearth this natural way of
breathing.

But when it becomes firmly established again, you'll be only too aware of
when you go off-track and revert to old ways. And you'll be able to correct
your breathing quickly and with confidence. Make a clean start. Relearn
physiologically sound, *normal* breathing.

*It's both unnatural as well as uncomfortable to think about your breathing. But
to ring the changes, breathing awareness is a prerequisite.*

The next crucial ingredient is making nose-breathing a *number one top
priority*. Remember the old saying – 'use it or lose it'; this is never more true
than of nose-breathing. Get all the help you can to restore this, if you do
have continuing problems. Your doctor can arrange a nasal CT scan (slightly

more expensive but much more revealing than an X-ray) to find out what is causing your nasal problems, and a visit to an Ear, Nose and Throat specialist might be a good option to have further checks. They are able to look up the nasal openings with a small light and check out what's wrong and show you what's going on up there – on a small screen, if you want!

Training yourself to nose-breathe may be uncomfortable at first because there is up to 50 per cent more resistance to the airflow compared to mouth-breathing. (Try switching from one to the other and feel the difference.) This takes some getting used to – but you may be very surprised at the pay-off.

> I'd been practising my new 'low slow nose-breathing' for about seven or eight days and suddenly I realised something amazing. I was smelling the chocolate I was mixing into a biscuit mixture. I hadn't had a sense of smell for about ten years. Can you imagine my delight? I was absolutely overjoyed. I walked round the house. I smelt the tang of some Brasso of all things – and the scent of some flowers. It was incredible. It comes and goes because I do have sinus problems – but from nasal washes and breathing through my nose I got such a wonderful result – after ten years.
> **Julia, 68**

Breathing retraining

The best place to start is to identify faulty breathing patterns. Place one hand on your stomach and the other on your upper chest. It's a good idea to keep your first finger resting on your collarbone and the other fingers resting lightly on your upper chest wall. As your collarbone stays relatively still during quiet breathing you can feel upper rib movement better.

- First, tune in to your breathing pattern. Are you most comfortable nose or mouth-breathing? Can you feel your upper chest moving at all?
- Try taking a deep breath. Did your stomach draw in or puff out? Did your upper chest lift up or stay still?

Chances are you took a *big* breath rather than a *deep* one and you led with your upper chest, puffing it up and stretching your upper chest wall while

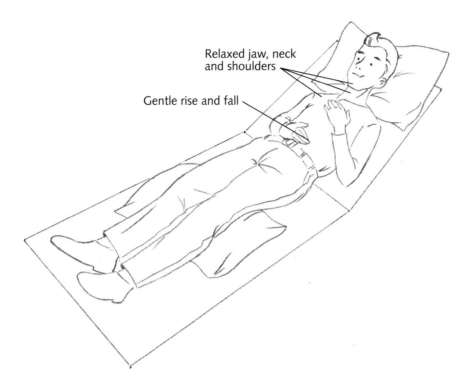

Relaxed jaw, neck and shoulders

Gentle rise and fall

sucking your stomach in (often the sort of breath taken when using your inhaler). This is 'reverse breathing' – a very common pattern in people with asthma. Did you mouth breathe as well?

Switch from nose- to mouth-breathing and feel the difference in both the *resistance* and *patterning*.

Check your breathing rate

Time your breathing for one minute (each breath in and out counts as 1).

Normal resting breathing rates are 10–14 per minute for adults, 15–25 for children and 25–50 for babies and toddlers.

Remember, when you are free of symptoms, habitually breathing too fast pushes too much air through the chest for the body to deal with. Carbon dioxide levels drop. Chronic hyperventilation and all its puzzling symptoms may become an added and *exhausting* problem.

Establishing nose/abdominal patterns

Learn to breathe low – relaxing your waist as you breathe in. A very good way to start is to clasp your hands on top of your head. This puts your upper chest muscles into 'neutral', making it harder for them to dominate your breathing.

Close your eyes and feel what's happening. Your abdominal wall should be gently expanding as you nose-breathe in, and elasticating back as you nose-breathe out. Relish the relaxed pause at the end of the out-breath – waiting for the in-breath to self-start naturally. This is one of the commonest obstacles to 'good breathing' – losing the knack of *breathing out fully* and missing out on the *relaxed* pause.

Once you have felt your waist expanding on the in-breath and relaxing back as you exhale, slowly lower your arms and see if you can keep breathing this way.

Most people find their trigger-happy upper chest muscles spring back into action straight away. It may take a lot of practice to change old habits, but prepare yourself for the long haul. It's worth it.

Learn to suppress upper chest breathing

When the motor cortex – the area in your brain that sends messages to muscles instructing them to work – starts habitually firing more messages to the upper chest muscles than to the diaphragm and lower chest muscles, this patterning becomes dominant. Stretch receptors in these muscles tend to put the body on 'red alert'. (After all, it is normal to upper chest-breathe in an emergency, or when you're under stress – the 'flight/fight' response.) Adrenalin surges into the blood stream and heart rate increases. Tension, sweaty palms, 'air hunger'. Sound familiar?

Concentrating on the out-breath and consciously relaxing your jaw, neck, shoulders and upper chest wall every time you breathe *out* during practice helps re-route the messages to your lower chest and away from the prevailing upper-chest pattern.

Remember upper-chest muscles are designed for short-term use only – 10 minutes here, half an hour there – not 24 hours a day!

Accelerated learning

A very helpful way to speed up learning to abdominal-nose breathe, bypassing your upper chest, is *biofeedback*. No complicated gadgetry is needed – only a 1 or 2 kilogram wheatpack or bag of rice (depending on your age/size).

Place the wheatpack on your stomach just below belt-buckle level so you can see as well as feel your diaphragm and abdominal wall muscles working together to produce relaxing, energy-efficient breathing.

After a few minutes of this, put the wheatpack on your upper chest and feel and see *no* movement as you abdominal-breathe.

If you have been on courses of oral steroids, the diaphragm may have weakened a little, and at first may feel a bit 'jumpy' as you start abdominal breathing. ('Staircase' or 'cogwheel' breathing is a popular phrase used to describe the jerky action of an exhausted diaphragm.) This just indicates your diaphragm muscle needs strengthening again. Practising with the wheatpack or perhaps Inspiratory Muscle Training (see page 58) is important for you to restore strength. (Check with your physiotherapist to see if IMT is a suitable option for you.)

Breathing Works breathing retraining programme

Consider this as a step-by-step plan to relearn normal breathing patterns. Begin retraining lying down at first so you can concentrate 100 per cent on doing it right. It's also a great opportunity to relax and take 'time out'.

Once the steps become familiar you can then start integrating these new patterns into daily life – sitting, standing, walking and talking, for instance.

The programme takes time and lots of repetition. Schedule two 10-minute sessions a day for two weeks. This is where commitment comes in.

Lying

Supported comfortably with pillows, start with the 'beach pose' – arms above your head to suppress upper chest movement and knees bent up to relax your stomach wall and lower back.

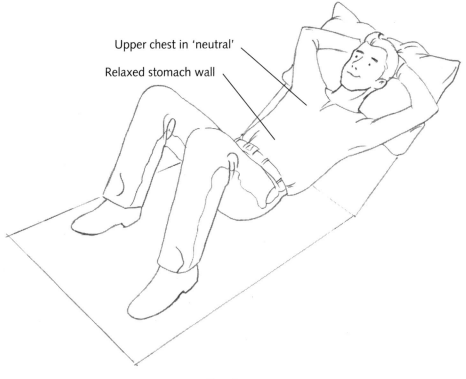

Upper chest in 'neutral'

Relaxed stomach wall

Beach pose

Tune into your nose-abdominal breathing pattern and relax at the end of each breath out, to slow your breathing rate.

Place the tip of your tongue behind your top front teeth to help relax your jaw and throat. It may help to time yourself at first by counting how many breaths a minute you are doing; 10–14 is the normal range to aim for. It's better, after a few practice sessions, to learn the 'feel' of breathing slower and lower rather than relying on clock-watching.

When you feel ready, slowly bring your arms down by your sides and stretch your legs out with a pillow under your knees.

Put the 1 or 2 kg wheatpack on your stomach for 4–5 minutes. Concentrate on the out-breath and the relaxed pause at the end of the breath out. It's more important for the weight to help you *breathe out* and relax. Avoid expanding your stomach wall too vigorously or pushing too far up when breathing in.

Take care not to 'hold' at the top of the in-breath.

Breathe out gently, relax and let the in-breath start itself. This 'letting go' can be a very strange feeling – but relax – your next in-breath *will* start all by itself with no prompting from you. Trust yourself!

Next, place the wheatpack on your upper chest for 4–5 minutes, concentrating on the stillness of your upper chest wall. Some people may find this very uncomfortable at first. Leave this part out if you do – and try again in a few days.

Try this if you feel wheezy or tight-chested to help relax chest, neck and jaw muscles. It's especially comforting if you warm up the wheatpack first.

An alternative is to place both hands lightly on your upper chest and focus on making sure your hands stay as still as possible.

In bed at night try nose/abdominal breathing while lying on your side. This is a great way to switch off tense muscles and help you sleep.

It's important to keep practising on a regular basis, even if you start to find it easier and feel better. At first it may make you experience uncomfortable feelings of 'air hunger'. This is a good sign, showing you are making progress. The breathing centres in your brain are being challenged to accept normal CO_2 levels again. Try hard – by swallowing hard – to prevent taking that longed-for 'big' breath.

At Breathing Works we use an oximeter – a small device that clips onto a finger, toe or earlobe – to measure oxygen saturations. This is measured as a percentage, normal being 95–98 per cent. You have a finite number of red blood cells and you can't load them with oxygen beyond 100 per cent saturation. (Many people with asthma, convinced they need more air, are very surprised to see they are absolutely fabulously 100 per cent saturated!) Having an oxygen saturation reading of 100 per cent is an indication that there may be too much CO_2 being blown out. This disturbs the body's acid balance, producing various physiological changes which lead to frightening symptoms.

Seeing for yourself that you do indeed have plenty of oxygen helps boost confidence – *you don't need to take that extra breath.*

It takes six to eight weeks of consistent awareness and practice for the new patterns to become strong and *established.*

> I kept up my practice religiously for about five days in a row. Honestly, I felt so much better after about two or three days – so of course I started forgetting about it or putting it off. But I started feeling bad again – I really had to put the practice in to get lasting results. It's the repetition that pays off.
> **Edward, 24**

Inspiratory Muscle Training (IMT)

Inspiratory (in-breath) muscles are prone to damage from over-stretching during acute asthma episodes. Anyone recovering from an acute attack will agree how tense and painful their chest muscles feel. This risk can be reduced by inspiratory muscle strengthening. IMT devices target the diaphragm. Asthma sufferers who have used these devices report reduced medication use and hospital admissions – with the added bonus that their exercise tolerance and fitness improved a great deal.

This type of training has a long history. Soldiers in the First World War recovering from lung damage from toxic gas inhalation were given thick wads of cotton wool to breathe into – to strengthen their chest muscles.

There are many types of IMTs on the market. One of the best-researched (and strongest – it's guaranteed to last five years) is the Powerbreathe – also known as 'dumbells for the lungs'. It was developed in the UK at the University of Birmingham Sports Medicine and Human Performance unit by Dr Alison McConnell, an exercise physiologist and keen sportswoman, who started her research on healthy older people experiencing breathlessness. The results were encouraging and she then found people with asthma benefited – as did top-flight athletes. Dr McConnell discovered that when athletes 'warmed up' their breathing muscles before competition as part of their general warm-up, they performed better and recovered more quickly. This was especially so for those with asthma.

After a really bad winter where I was plagued with chest infections and worsening asthma, I got into a real cycle of decline! I lost a lot of fitness and found I couldn't mow the lawns or do things I normally could. I had repeat courses of prednisone, antibiotics and felt worse. I gained weight and couldn't exercise because of shortness of breath, which scared me a bit. I ended up being sent to a chest specialist. She suggested some breathing re-education while she tinkered with my medications. I was a shocker – shoulder muscles like rocks and so locked into breathing high into my chest. I couldn't believe it when it was pointed out. I was totally unaware of my neck and chest. My breathing rate was 24 breaths a minute. Twice as fast as normal. My peak flow was 340 – lower than it should be. I was encouraged to use a Powerbreathe which was easy once I got the knack. It only took a couple of minutes morning and evening so it wasn't a chore. I felt an enormous improvement within two weeks. My peak flow went up to 370. My Ventolin consumption went right down too. After eight weeks I had a peak flow of 450. The breathing retraining and diaphragm strengthening helped me turn a corner. In all my years as an asthmatic – 30-odd years – I had never received any help with breathing; the emphasis was always on medication.

I know I can't do without my puffers – and I know breathing better doesn't 'cure' my asthma – but my quality of life has improved out of sight. I can exercise comfortably, I'm much fitter, my weight has dropped – and I enjoy mowing the lawn again. **Molly, 47**

Try this

Putting it all together

While this daily basic groundwork to reclaim energy-efficient breathing is being practised, try these tips for integrating good breathing patterns into your daily life:

- Practise while sitting as well as standing. Clasping your hands behind you helps release shoulder and neck tension and brings the diaphragm into action.

- Watch out for 'chest bracing' – the old habit of hyperinflating the upper chest and holding in too much air.
- Every hour, on the hour STOP: check your chest, DROP: shoulders loose and down, FLOP: release tension in your whole body (jaw, small of your back, legs and hands).
- Concentrate on your breathing – nose/low/slow for a minute or two – then *forget about your breathing*. Don't think about it all the time. As your breathing patterns improve there will be less need to check your chest so often.
- Use visual cues to help remind yourself to nose breathe and drop your shoulders – e.g. bright stickers on your computer, fridge, TV, dashboard of the car.

After chest infections, colds or asthma episodes go back to 'start' and increase your daily practice again.

- Stressful events can be responsible for causing the upper chest to leap into action again, often with wheezing. Concentrating on physical coping skills helps you unwind – both in mind and body.
- Don't be a martyr if you feel unwell. Take time out and nourish your airways and yourself with relaxed and balanced breathing.
- When you become really good at low/slow/nose-breathing you may find yourself comfortably breathing as low as 6-10 breaths per minute. This shows you have switched on your 'relaxation response', which is the best drug-free weapon in your armoury to combat asthma.
- Remember that breathing is naturally chaotic during asthma attacks. Use Rest Positions (see page 38) to help conserve energy. Check your breathing patterns when the attack is over. Increased medications – especially relievers – can lead to 'speediness'. Make sure your upper chest hasn't joined in.
- Practise reading aloud and check you are using abdominal breaths – not upper chest heaves – while talking. People whose jobs involve talking a lot need to pay special attention to this.
- Try a course of IMT – check with your physiotherapist.

To sum up: If your breathing goes high in your chest with sighs, breathe yourself gently down and out of trouble. *When in doubt, breathe out*.

The Buteyko Method

Anyone who has asthma or who has a child with asthma wants to find out as much as they can about other ways of approaching this disorder. The Buteyko Method has created a lot of interest, particularly in Western countries such as the UK, Australia and New Zealand. Devised by Dr Konstantin Buteyko in Russia in the 1960s, the method was used as one of many options in asthma treatment by physiotherapists there. Unfortunately many Western Buteyko practitioners have no medical training. **If you decide to use this method, then make sure you choose a practitioner with a medical background.**

The key features of the method include:

• Encouraging very shallow breathing – *hypo*ventilation – to counter *hyper*ventilation, which is so common in people with asthma. Specific breathing techniques are taught to be carried out for 20 minutes twice a day.

• Use of a 'control pause' where the out-breath is held until there is a distinct sensation of slight lack of air. Breathing must remain shallow, and the pause must not be followed by a deep breath.

• First-aid use of a 'maximum pause' where the out-breath is held until moderate discomfort is felt, resuming breathing without losing control of the shallow pattern.

Warning: Anyone with lung, heart or kidney disease, hypertension, epilepsy or diabetes should use the 'maximum pause' with caution. Similar to re-breathing CO_2 from a paper bag, prolonged breath-holding may cause oxygen levels to drop beyond safe levels. If you suffer from the above diseases you may already have lowered oxygen levels, or compromise your diseased or distressed organs by inflicting a sudden drop in oxygen, or hypoxaemia. *An oximeter (a small portable device to measure blood oxygen saturations) should always be used during supervised training sessions.*

Comment

The Buteyko Method suits some people very well, particularly if they have anxieties over taking medication, and have carried out all the other environmental control, dietary and fitness advice offered by free Asthma Education programmes. Some doctors have become very wary of the method after children in their care have ended up in hospital with severe attacks after 'preventer' dose reduction without their knowledge. But most family doctors will support one's rights to choose alternative therapies as long as they are kept informed (a common courtesy).

CHAPTER 8

Posture and body mechanics

Many of us have developed ways of using our bodies that affect the way we breathe. As a result this has a direct effect on our health.

> After a breathing retraining session last year, I gained an appreciation of the breathing process and a sense of reassurance that I could do something about it and that I didn't have to be crippled by asthma. I learnt that my breathing pattern was largely based upon not 'letting the air out'; this revelation was quite a surprise to me. I just didn't realise that when I couldn't get any air it was because I hadn't let the previous breath out. However, I was still constrained by my faulty body awareness in which I didn't recognise when I was holding my breath, nor was I aware of the held muscle tension that caused me to brace my chest and dramatically restrict the use of my diaphragm when breathing. I have been unconsciously breathing that way all of my life. Over the last ten months or so I have investigated a number of therapies to help with this and I'm slowly becoming aware of the tension-holding patterns that need to be released in order to improve my breathing.
>
> I think that for people who suffer 'my kind' of asthma, poor breathing becomes a learned response to stressful situations, even though their asthma may have initially begun years before through allergy, virus or whatever. I know now that learning to breathe properly and becoming aware of held tensions in order to release them is crucial to restoring good breathing. **Lewis, 39**

Why is good posture so important?

Good posture maintains health and wellbeing, ensures stress-free movements and energy-efficient breathing patterns, and it looks good.

Posture refers to the body's alignment and positioning with respect to the force of gravity. Whether we are standing, sitting or lying down, gravity exerts a force on our joints, ligaments and muscles. Good posture ensures these structures are not over-stressed.

An ideal posture is to follow a plumb-line from the earlobe to the back of your collarbone, through the tip of the shoulder joint to the centre of the hip, to the outside bump of the ankle. The centre of the knee is slightly behind that line. We refer to this as neutral alignment.

Ideally, from a back view the spine and legs should be straight. With this ideal, neutral alignment the body weight is balanced about the spine, allowing minimal muscular effort and avoiding excess stress on the joints, discs and ligaments.

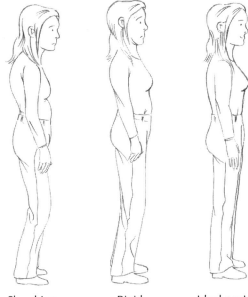

Slouching   Rigid   Ideal posture

Breathing and movement

Physical awareness

Body mechanics refers to the way we position our body to carry out movement – activities such as pushing, lifting or carrying. And just like good static posture, 'good' body mechanics will allow one to work and play more efficiently and with less stress on any one body part.

Good breathing works to transmit forces efficiently through the body. With each inhalation and exhalation the body moves up and down, forwards and backwards, in and out. The breath works in combination with the body, allowing energy-efficient movements to occur.

Poor posture

An over-corrected posture often leads to over-inflated lungs, giving the appearance of a puffed-up chest. As a result, the upper body becomes tense and the upper chest and neck muscles are used as the main breathing muscles.

Try tightening every muscle in your body, pull your tummy in and puff your chest out as if you are an Olympic weightlifter. Now take a breath into the upper chest, hold it there. Now breathe on top of this.

Is it harder to breathe? How do you feel?

Muscles that are too tight will affect your ability to breathe effectively and function effectively.

The slouched posture is also inefficient: muscle tone is poor and this reflects in the posture; breathing is weak. Try sitting in a chair, then let your body slouch. Come on, drop those shoulders forwards, bend over. Now feel your breathing pattern. What does this feel like? Has your breathing changed?

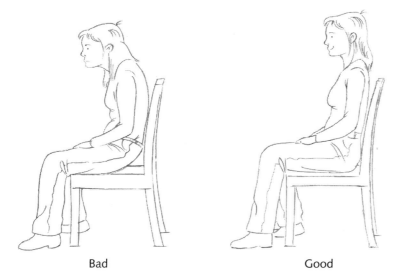

Bad   Good

This posture resembles a sagging cardboard box. Rounded shoulders restrict the ribcage movement and poor breathing will occur. A sagging belly and slouched posture all contribute to ineffective breathing.

Sitting is when most of us get into trouble with poor postural habits, especially when driving or using a computer. How often have you found yourself with your nose almost touching your computer screen?

The body has a habit of following our head, so as we become engrossed in our work, our head moves forward, shoulders become rounded, our spine curves and our breathing will change to perhaps mouth and certainly upper chest.

Ideally, while sitting, the S-shaped curvature of the spine that is characteristic of good standing posture should be maintained.

Effect of poor posture on asthma

The poor postures described above are commonly found amongst people who have asthma. These postures quickly become the norm and are reinforced by poor upper chest breathing patterns. As we have seen, this all too quickly becomes a vicious cycle reinforcing breathing pattern disorders, leading to over-breathing, muscle fatigue, general fatigue, and further susceptibility to our asthma and allergies.

The following exercises are designed to:

- improve your posture,
- maintain good, healthy breathing patterns,
- strengthen the trunk for neutral stability.

Tune into your body: awareness is the key

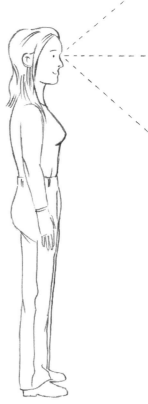

Awareness of good posture is the first step to breaking old, poor, postural habits and reducing stress and strain on your spine.

Exercise 1: Check your posture

Stand in your natural posture and relax. In this relaxed position, where are your eyes looking? To the horizon, up in the air or down at the ground? If your posture is straight and head position correct, your eyes should be looking down at approximately 45 degrees. Anything above this means that your head is poking forwards and upwards – a very common problem in today's society.

Check yourself in a full-length mirror. Look side-on to see how you compare with the picture.

Finding neutral

The latest gym lingo is to talk about the 'core position'. What they are talking about is your neutral alignment. Core stability refers to stabilising the trunk region by strengthening some of the deep abdominal muscles.

Your aim is to recognise what neutral alignment looks and feels like in your body. You should be able to move into neutral alignment while sitting, standing and moving. Neutral alignment is the position in which the spine is best equipped to deal with external stress and strain.

Exercise 2: Finding neutral in lying

1. Lie on your back with your knees bent and feet flat on the ground. Firstly become aware of your abdomen (belly), noticing how it moves when you breathe in and out. See if it is tense or loose.

Try tensing your belly by pulling it in towards the floor. Now release.

If your breathing is not free and flowing when you do these exercises, return to Chapter 7 and try the effective breathing exercises before progressing.

2. While lying, firstly try what is called a pelvic tilt. To do this, gently rock your pelvis up towards the ceiling, feeling your spine flatten, then rock it back towards the floor, feeling your spine arch. Now let go. Repeat, aiming for a rhythmical rock. This time, as you rock tilt your pelvis towards the floor and breathe in. As you tilt your pelvis to the ceiling breathe out. Feel the freedom of movement in this area; feel your abdomen open as you tilt to the floor and breathe in and close as you tilt up and breathe out.

3. Now focus on your pelvic floor. The pelvic floor runs from the tip of your pubic bone to your coccyx (tailbone), and encompasses all the muscles and tissues in between. Try to identify these muscles by drawing them up between your legs.

Women: imagine drawing up your vagina and rectum as if stopping the flow of urine mid-stream; now release. Try this a few times.

Men: imagine you are standing over a barbed-wire fence; you don't want your testicles to be caught, so draw your testicles up. Feel the sensation of drawing up between your legs; now release. Try this a few times.

After all – this is the bottom of the cardboard box and you cannot afford the base to be saggy!

Now let's try and combine both sensations, remembering to breathe in when you tilt your pelvis down toward the floor and to breathe out when you tilt towards the ceiling. While tilting your pelvis towards the ceiling, gently draw up your pelvic floor and breathe out. Now release, tilting back as you breathe in. Repeat this a few times until it is a rhythmical, flowing movement.

This time concentrate on your lower abdomen, gently tightening it as you tilt to the ceiling. Repeat this exercise four times, drawing up for a hold of four seconds.

The neutral position is found when the pelvis comes to rest in the mid-line. This is the mid position between the extremes of the pelvic movement.

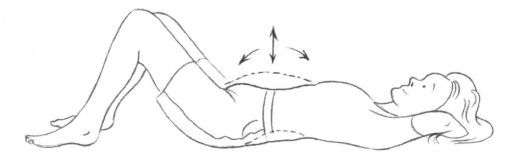

Exercise 3: Progress to neutral while sitting

The first step is to identify your seat bones – the ischial tuberosities. To do this, place your hands under your bottom and rock backwards and forwards on your hands in the chair. At the point of most pressure on your hands stop and take your hands away: maintain this position, as this should be optimum pelvic-neutral.

If you have difficulty finding pelvic-neutral, rock your pelvis backwards and forwards and rest in between.

Exercise 4: Neutral in standing

Work between the two postures of standing from extremely erect to slouching (see page 64); gently work your way into the neutral of these two postures. Try to mimic the plumb-line as much as possible – roll your shoulders backwards and forwards to find the in-between.

Now open your chest, making it as wide across as you can with the least effort; don't let those shoulders rise up, and don't forget to breathe.

Rock your pelvis – find pelvic-neutral – tuck an imaginary tail between your legs and release.

Now imagine a string attached to your head; let this string pull you up and elongate you, allowing your body to elongate with you, standing tall but with ease and grace. While holding this position – staying elongated – breathe out, ensuring your tongue, jaw, shoulders and pelvic floor are all relaxed.

Notice how you feel. If you increase awareness of your body and posture, with time this will become your pattern automatically; you will need to be diligent initially, reminding yourself throughout the day.

Exercise 5: Lower abdominals

This is aimed at strengthening the lower abdominal muscles. These muscles we know are vital for trunk stability and help form part of the abdominal brace that enables good, efficient breathing patterns. They work to maintain body-neutral throughout movement. If we lose this stability what results is muscle imbalance, leading to stress and strain being placed upon joints and supporting soft tissues.

Note: Holding the abdominals in a constant state of tension, i.e. continually holding in your belly, can actually weaken the muscles. It also adds to tension and stiffness in the lower back.

In effective breathing postures the abdominals move with each breath, swelling the belly with the breath in, and flattening with the breath out. This does not of course mean letting it all hang out – it means allowing your abdomen to move as it should with each effective breath and at the same time maintaining truly good postures.

Try to identify the deep muscles involved in stabilising the trunk. Lie with your knees bent; a good way to find these muscles is to place your fingers on the inside area of your hip bones and cough: the muscles that pop up are your internal oblique muscles and transversus abdominis.

The aim of this exercise is to try to activate these muscles, as they are vital for trunk and abdominal stability.

Now find pelvic-neutral using the pelvic floor exercise above. Holding gently in pelvic-neutral, draw the tissues up in the pelvic region and gently tighten the lower deep abdominal muscle – *remember to breathe*. You should be able to maintain nose-belly breathing. Hold and release. Repeat four times.

To advance, continue as above – it is essential to keep your back flat on the floor during this exercise. Gently tightening the deep abdominal muscle – and still breathing – keeping your back on the ground, slowly lift one leg to 90°. Do not lift your back. BREATHE and then slowly let your leg return to the ground – still not lifting your back and keeping breathing. Repeat four times with each leg.

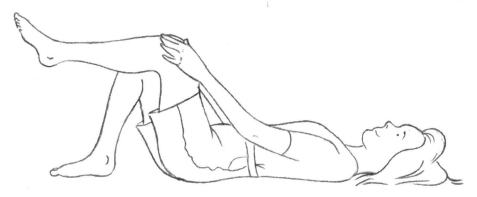

A rule of thumb

- Inhalation leads to arching (extension) of the spine.
- Exhalation leads to flattening (flexion) of the spine.
- Inhalation leads to the opening of the arms out from the body.
- Exhalation leads to the closing of the arms across the body.

If you practise the correct postures in neutral enough times, eventually your muscular memory will reprogramme these patterns and they will become natural. Remember, it takes six weeks to reprogramme muscular patterns.

CHAPTER 9

Breathing and exercise

Exercise is good for us: the benefits are well documented. For people with asthma physical activity is very important. When you are active you usually find you have less asthma and cope better.

What happens to our breathing during exercise?

- As we start to exercise breathing becomes deeper and faster, increasing to up to 50 breaths a minute.
- Greater amounts of oxygen are required to reach the muscles and tissues. Larger volumes of air are moved. With exercise the demand on the lungs increases 20-fold. Compare this to that of the heart, which only increases six-fold.
- Our relaxed pause phase is lost.
- We see the upper chest and often mouth-breathing patterns emerge. Different muscle groups are called upon to work. The neck and shoulder muscles are called upon to help with breathing in, and the trunk and abdominal muscles are called upon to help when we breathe out.

All this is totally normal.

Asthma is the most common cause of exercise-induced shortness of breath – but it is certainly not the only cause. Other factors can lead to shortness of breath, such as general and specific fitness levels, over-breathing and hyperventilation.

The stronger the respiratory muscles the less oxygen they require so they will literally steal less from other muscles in the body. If they are weak this leads to a cycle such as that shown on the next page.

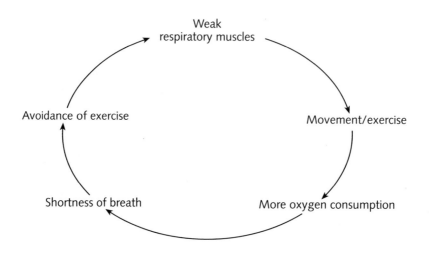

Tip number 1

Good, strong inspiratory muscles help oxygen efficiency and energy levels (see inspiratory muscle training, page 58).

Remember that shortness of breath is not always harmful but merely an indication to slow down and let the body recover.

Tip number 2

Exercise must be balanced with bouts of rest and recovery.

Exercise-induced asthma

Exercise-induced asthma may be the only form of asthma an individual experiences. It is too easy to attribute symptoms to other causes, e.g. age, lack of fitness or laziness. A person may be unaware they suffer from asthma, but will often suffer from symptoms during a respiratory tract infection or sinusitis. If you do experience signs and symptoms with exercise take notice, since it may be exercise-induced asthma.

The condition can affect people of any age and be brought on by any type of exercise; however there are some sports and forms of exercise that are more common causes than others. It is not restricted to just exercise. We should rename it activity-induced asthma, as it can also apply to lifestyle activities such as playing with children, housework and sexual activity.

How do I know if I have exercise-induced asthma?

It is characterised by breathlessness, wheezing, a tight chest, coughing, shortness of breath and/or chest tightness. Less common symptoms include stomachache, headache, fatigue, muscle cramps, chest pain and chest discomfort. Symptoms can occur at the beginning of and during exercise, although commonly in exercise-induced asthma symptoms will occur within one minute of ceasing exercise.

If you have symptoms more than three times a week your asthma is not well managed. Many people get wheezy with exercise; this is also a sign of asthma not being well controlled, so see your GP or a specialist for a review or for an assessment.

Exercise phases and related breathing cycles

At the beginning of exercise breathing is larger and faster. This leads to a drop in CO_2 and normal hyperventilation occurs, which may cause symptoms by triggering broncho-constriction or exercise-induced asthma.

Approximately 10–15 minutes into exercise, metabolic changes have taken effect as a result and CO_2 is produced. Increased CO_2 can make a bad breather feel better, i.e. it is common for many bad breathers to comment that they feel better 10–15 minutes into exercise.

At the end of exercise, if you continue to over-breathe this can lead to CO_2 depletion again and the signs and symptoms of over-breathing (hyperventilation) occur, leading to broncho-spasm and asthma.

High-triggering activities

Exercise-induced asthma has been recognised to occur under certain circumstances and is more prevalent during certain activities.

- Sustained activities during which large volumes of air are moved quickly over time, such as long-distance running, cycling, rowing, soccer, basketball and rugby.
- Activities associated with cool dry climates, e.g. ice-skating, ice hockey, etc.
- Activities at high altitude, especially if the weather is cool and dry, e.g. cross-country skiing.

Low-triggering activities

- Activities that are more stop-start, such as tennis, golf, karate, boxing and sprinting.
- Activities at sub-maximal levels, such as walking, tramping, yoga and martial arts.
- Swimming is often encouraged, as this is one sport where breathing patterns are considered important, and the warm, humid air is also thought to help. It is common for bad breathers to comment they find swimming difficult – this is a good indicator they are unaware of the correct breathing patterns. Unfortunately chlorinated pools may irritate nasal sinuses and trigger symptoms.

What causes exercise-induced asthma?

The cause of exercise-induced asthma is unknown, but there are two theories.

1. Water loss theory

Over-breathing (hyperventilation) leads to loss of water in the lining in the upper airways – this causes changes in cell pH (acid-alkaline balance) and cell temperature, which as a result cause broncho-constriction.

Another factor is mouth-breathing. With increased demand we normally use our mouths; the air is unfiltered and dry, and the upper airway will contribute water vapour in an attempt to moisten the air. This causes imbalances in the airway surface liquid – which leads to broncho-constriction.

2. Respiratory heat exchange theory

Loss of heat in the airways during and post exercise causes the bronchial vessels to swell to rewarm the airway lining. This causes airway narrowing, which releases more fluid into the tissue, resulting in broncho-constriction.

Factors contributing to exercise-induced asthma

- poor breathing patterns
- cold, dry air – this irritates already inflamed airways
- long periods of exercise, e.g. long-distance running

- pollens for allergic individuals
- air pollutants, e.g. tobacco smoke, exhaust fumes
- pre-existing upper respiratory tract infection, sinus infection or bronchitis
- exercise using either the legs or arms is less likely to induce an attack, e.g. cycling is better than exercises that use the whole body, such as running

Preventative strategies

- Practise good breathing patterns at rest and during exercise
- Do inspiratory muscle training
- Warming up before exercise or playing games can be useful; warm up at approximately 80 per cent of maximal cardiac output. Several 30-second sprints at sub-maximal cardiac levels over 5–10 minutes can protect the lungs, e.g. two minutes' exercise, then rest and recover, repeat four times. Skipping, running on the spot and jogging are good warm-up exercises.
- Exercise in warm, humid conditions
- Take reliever medication prior to sport
- Choose the right type of exercise, e.g. swimming, karate
- Maintain general fitness levels
- Other important factors for physiological balance are good sleep and a healthy diet. SLEEP WELL – EAT WELL – BREATHE WELL
- Choose stop-start activities
- When it's cold, wear a thin, warm scarf loosely around your face, a face-mask or a ski mask; these help to warm and moisten cool, dry air
- Exercise in non-irritant environments, e.g. avoid polluted, pollen-laden or cold environments.

Exercise-induced hyperventilation

Over-breathing can also lead to the sensation of shortness of breath; however this can occur in the absence of broncho-spasm – it is all too common for people to seek treatment thinking they have exercise-induced asthma when it may not be – it could be exercise-induced hyperventilation.

It is important to remember hyperventilation can trigger broncho-spasm.

I could not believe it: I had finally achieved my dream of top-class rugby and then asthma hit – or so I thought. On bad days I would have run literally two lengths of the field and I would get chest pain and shortness of breath – I just could not get a satisfying breath. To be honest it terrified me. How was I going to last a full game? Let alone the gruelling season. All I had worked for was gone.

Luckily my GP was onto it and referred me to a breathing specialist who worked out that the new training regime and weights programme I had been on had led to over-development in my upper body – I must admit I was looking a little like Charles Atlas. This posture I had developed had caused me to hyperinflate – over-breathe. I was already so puffed up that with added exertion I literally couldn't breathe in any more. I misread this 'air hunger feeling' as not enough, when in actual fact it was too much. I now breathe well through a game – shortness of breath is under control – and I have learnt that what counts is my breathing control and good patterns. My posture is much more balanced and I feel great – no puffers – no asthma. **John, 28**

Studies carried out in the USA have revealed the high incidence of children who use inhalers unnecessarily. People know that asthma is the most common cause of exercise-induced shortness of breath, so it is understandable that asthma is diagnosed. Studies have shown that some children who were initially diagnosed with asthma were in fact hyperventilating with exertion; the symptoms presented were similar to asthma, i.e. shortness of breath and tight chests. In exercise-induced hyperventilation people breathe faster than they need to and they experience difficulty breathing – often this is a normal response to a normal level of discomfort, especially if we have pushed ourselves too hard in exercise or our pattern has become one of over-breathing and hyperinflation. Some feel 'air hunger'. It is also evident in the gym culture, where people who exercise regularly often complain of shortness of breath that is disproportionate to their fitness levels. Commonly the cause is over-breathing – hyperinflation – in conjunction with a splinted diaphragm (held tense by the continuous pulling in of the belly) in an attempt to reach what the gym culture terms 'core stability'.

Mouth-chest breathing is a clear sign; this quickly leads to hyperinflation and common sensations of 'air hunger' and chest pain. Breathing retraining and inspiratory muscle training has been shown to be of vital importance to correct exercise-induced hyperventilation.

Exercise-induced asthma (EIA) or exercise-induced hyperventilation (EIH)?

	EIA	EIH
Medication	Will respond	Will not respond
Peak Expiratory Flow Rate (PEFR) measures	Will drop by up to 20 per cent post exercise	No change
	Broncho-spasm is the problem	Hyper-inflation is the problem
	Inflamed airways is the problem	Low CO_2 is the problem

Note: Low CO_2 and rapid breathing can cause broncho-spasm.

Good breathing patterns during exercise

Everyone, especially people with exercise-induced asthma, need to learn to incorporate breathing techniques into their training routines.

Use abdominal breathing before moving to higher chest breathing (your reserve tank!), along with comfortable nose-breathing. This is the most effective way to breathe when you exercise. With heavy exercise, of course, it is normal to mouth-breathe.

Diaphragmatic breathing combined with chest- and proper nose-breathing is the simplest and most effective way to breathe when you exercise.

Start initially with basic breathing regimes at rest (see Chapter 7) and nasal breathing (see page 51). Then begin to incorporate these regimes into your sport. Start with breathing and rhythm. Breathing rhythms during walking/stair climbing/running should be:

- two steps, breathe in,
- three steps, breathe out.

Ratios can be adapted to suit fitness levels, the intensity of the exercise or the steepness of the stairs/hills.

It may be helpful to start out with your hands loosely clasped behind your back, to help relax and soften tense shoulders. Release when a rhythm is established and enjoy relaxed arm swings. It is easy to do this when playing stop-start sports, for example:

- In tennis, focus on breathing between bouts and incorporate it into your game – remember the Monica Seles grunt. Martina Navratilova was famous for nose-breathing throughout her games.
- At golf, when you hit the ball use your breathing to help with concentration, e.g. breathe in as you swing back, breathe out 1, 2, 3, as you swing forward and hit the ball. Relaxed breathing in-between holes can help calm any performance nerves.

It is vital after sport to slow down your breathing gradually and in a controlled manner – the aim is to get back to nose-diaphragm breathing.

If you practise exercises such as yoga, t'ai chi, Pilates, Feldenkrais or martial arts remember that their breathing techniques are exercises that are related to their philosophies. It is important to return to usual, relaxed breathing after these exercise sessions.

Chapter 10

Stretches and movement

It feels so good to stretch my chest, neck and shoulder muscles. After doing the Breathing Works exercise routine I feel a weight literally lift off my chest, the suffocating feeling goes. I can breathe easy. I do have to keep the exercises up, though. I have a very busy job and at the end of a busy week I'm a little tense – my muscles are tense and I notice my breathing is faster with less pause phase. After the stretches I feel much better. **Tony, 42**

Stretching and movement reduces muscle tension and prevents poor postures from occurring. It expands our awareness of our body, increases our circulation, improves our body mechanics and posture, and balances our muscles to create a body able to function efficiently.

As we have seen, poor breathing patterns can lead to poor postures and vice versa. The following are stretches to avoid such postures and maintain muscles in their optimum, neutral state for healthy, efficient breathing. Our goal is to:

- Relax tense muscles of the neck, shoulder region and trunk,
- Mobilise the spine and ribcage,
- Maintain good movement of the body and breathing structures.

Exercises for children under ten

The most vital thing for children is to keep the chest open, to nose-belly breathe and to avoid poor postures. If this can be programmed in from an early age the children will benefit enormously.

Far too often we see children breathing though their mouths, with shoulders around their ears and sitting hunched up – this is quite wrong and leads to poor health. Regular routines are essential.

Talking to Alex ($9^1/_2$, life-long asthma, main allergens are cats, dust mites and exercise) after three breathing sessions and three months of breathing practice.

Q: *Alex, what have you noticed since you have been doing breathing exercises?*
A: My nose is a lot clearer. I can hold my breath longer. I find it easier to run around and play sport. I can't remember what it's like to be short of breath – I haven't been ill for a long time. I don't wake up in the middle of the night coughing any more. I cough less when I'm ill; I also don't stop and cough in the middle of laughing.
Sue, Alex's mother: The main thing is Alex is more aware of his breathing. For example, two weeks ago Alex started coughing, I encouraged him to focus on his breathing and to keep his fluids up. Which he did, normally he would cough constantly, further irritating the airways, and end up on a nebuliser. So this time we didn't get to that next stage. He had a day of rest, and believe it or not the following day he played in the school hockey match. I think that is what this is about – Alex is now at the age I feel he can take control for himself. He has some tools to work with. His energy is better and his nose is clearer.

Hot Tip 1. Breathe in, breathe out and relax

Aim for a controlled exhalation followed by a relaxed pause. This is often the reverse for people with asthma, especially children, who tend to puff up their upper chests like a balloon that is about to burst. Our lungs should only be one-third full for effective breathing, the reserve is for exercise or strenuous activities. Try the following exercises and have fun!

- Try blowing up balloons, blowing bubbles or bubble gum – when it's time to breathe in make sure it is nose-abdomen, and ensure all the air is blown out gently. Do not force the breath out.
- Practise blowing a piece of paper: hold the paper in your fingers or let the child do this themselves and ask them to blow in a steady and continuous manner. Then make it a little more challenging by timing how long they can blow out before they literally run out of puff.

- Blow a ping-pong ball across the table in a controlled pattern; make it a game to see who can blow it in a straight line and encourage them to blow through pursed lips as this will prevent irritation to the airway, which will occur if all the air is huffed out at once in a forced manner.
- Imitate Gollum in *The Lord of the Rings*: repeat the phrase 'my precioussssssss', emphasising the 's'.

Hot Tip 2. The nose is vital

Exercises to encourage nose-breathing:

- Open your eyes as wide as you can and 'make a face' with your hands (see picture). With fingers on your cheekbones and on your forehead, stretch open your eyes and nostrils. This stretch will open up your sinuses and the bones around this area. These often become tense and tight, making nose-breathing difficult. While you are doing this gently close your mouth and try to nose-breathe; it may be hard at first but continue until you have an even flow of air through your nose.

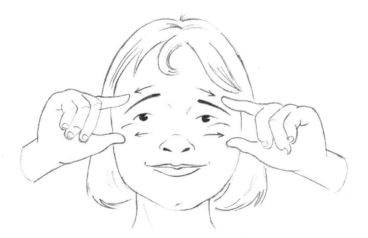

- Try sucking on a lollipop using 'no hands'. Keeping the lollipop in your mouth, gently focus on nose-breathing. (A hard sweet or a large peppermint can also be used.) This keeps the tongue gently on the roof of the mouth where it should normally sit, allowing relaxation of the jaw and easy airflow through the sinuses.

- Nasal strips are readily available from the chemist; use these for a couple of days to assist nasal air entry. They are ideal when sleeping.
- Practise drinking through a straw; when it is time to breathe use the nose.

Hot Tip 3. Diaphragm breathing and strength are vital for endurance

Exercises for strong belly-breathing patterns:

- This exercise can be done while watching television, or before relaxed breathing at night. Find a weight, preferably 1 kg initially – a bag of rice is ideal. While lying with your knees bent, place the weight on your abdomen around the area of your bellybutton. Breathe out of your mouth; relax. Now breathing in through your nose and belly, focus on the weight and gently lift it (just gently; a large volume of air is not what you want). When you feel the rhythm is flowing, breathe in and out of your nose. Practise twice a day for five minutes for a week. After a week progress to two kg for two weeks, twice daily for five minutes. Your diaphragm pattern should be strengthening by now. For the next three weeks once a day is adequate; then after this three to four times a week as in any exercise routine.

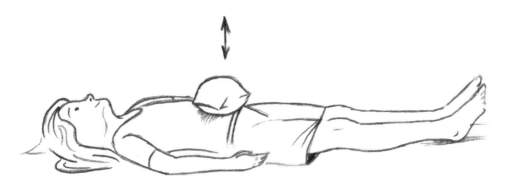

- Narrow tubes will increase the resistance of breathing; this works the breathing-in muscles harder, so you could practise this by blowing through a straw to increase resistance, or using a wind instrument such as a recorder.
- There are also specific devices designed for strengthening the inspiratory muscles (see page 58).

Hot Tip 4. Activity must be balanced with rest

This exercise encourages a relaxed pause phase, leading to relaxed, healthy breathing.

Exercises for relaxation:

- Gently breathe in and out, pausing at the end of the out-breath. Breathe in when you feel you need to; repeat, and this time try to hang on for a little longer before taking in your next breath.
- Sleep is vital for the balance of the body. Prior to sleep it is helpful to do some quiet, relaxed breathing.

For younger children it is often easier to build the exercises into a game, or to use the same routine on a regular basis. The following movements are specifically for good spinal, chest and breathing muscle health.

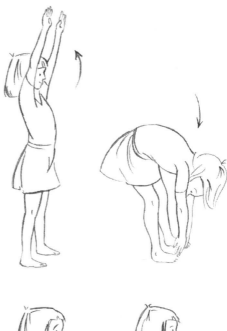

- Breathe in and stretch all the way up to the ceiling, then blow out with all your might and touch your toes.

- While standing, keep your lower body still; roll your shoulders backwards, breathing in as you do so. As you breathe out, encourage a 'hmmmm' sound with the breath.

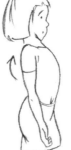
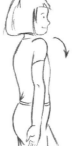

- While standing, move your arms from side to side – breathing in as you go to the left and out as you go to the right. This could be done while playing with a golf club, cricket bat or baseball bat.

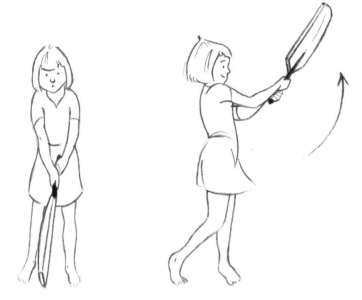

- To open the chest wall lean back over the sofa, beanbag or Swiss ball while breathing into your belly through your nose, low and slow. Or lie on your stomach while watching television – you must do this for at least half an hour.

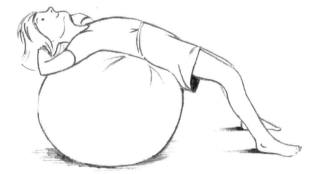

All these exercises can be used by adults.

Teenagers and adults

These four stretches are essential to maintain a mobile chest wall.

Stretch 1: Scalenes

While standing against a wall breathe out, placing your hand on your opposite shoulder and holding. (This is to stabilise the point at which the muscle joins the first rib.) Then breathe in and gently stretch your neck to the opposite side. Try to keep your head still as you breathe out. Hold and return to neutral.

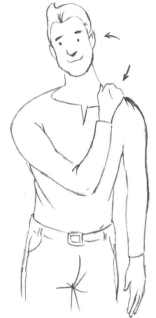

Repeat, but this time gently nod your head forward and breathe in; stretch to the opposite side and breathe out. Return to normal.

Take a step forwards and gently tilt your head backwards and stretch to the opposite side.

Repeat the above using the opposite side of the body.

Stretch 2: Sternocleidomastoids

Stand against the wall again. Gently nod your head using the top of the neck (just like you are making a very subtle bid in an auction) and hold; now, with the most minimal of movements turn your head to one side, hold, making sure you are breathing. Finish with a side bend to the top of the neck on the opposite side, i.e. bring your ear to your shoulder.

Stretch 3: Pectoralis major and minor

These chest muscles commonly get tight, causing shoulders to turn inwards, resulting in ineffective breathing patterns. Sitting on a chair, with your back straight, chin tucked in and feet flat on the ground, place your hands at either end of a piece of rope or belt (sit straight with your arms far enough apart so that you can stretch them above your head).

Breathe in, and with your arms straight lift them up and over your head without bringing your neck forwards; bring the rope behind you, breathe out and feel the stretch; breathe in and return to the resting position and breathe out. Repeat four times.

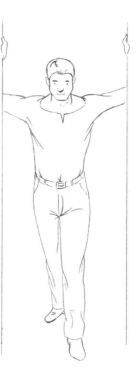

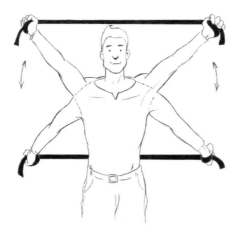

While standing, place your elbows at shoulder height in a doorway. Breathe in and stretch, breathe out.

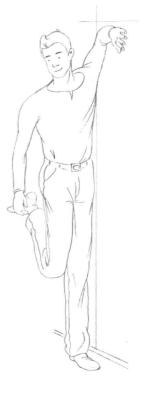

Stretch 4: Iliopsoas/hamstrings

While standing hold the wall for support; bend your knee backwards, holding your ankle with your hand and keeping your hip straight, lean forwards and feel a stretch to the front of your hip and thigh. Repeat with the other leg.

The Breathing Works 'Fab Four'

Four minutes a day keeps bad breathing away. The following stretches are quick and easy and they can be done while watching television, at the traffic lights, while cleaning your teeth, or in the office. They have been designed to keep the upper body, head and jaw mobile and tension-free.

Stretch 1: Chin tuck

While standing or sitting, keeping your chin parallel with the floor, pull your chin back towards your neck; hold and release. Practise this exercise while against a wall so you can feel the sensation of the stretch. Imagine a book under your chin; now glide your chin backwards along the book, stretching up the back of the neck. Or imagine a string is attached to your head; let this string pull you up from the back of the neck and let it elongate you. This stretch releases tension at the back of the neck and also helps with postural alignment.

Stretch 2: Tongue stretch

Open your mouth and stretch your tongue out as far as you can, trying to touch the tip of your chin, then relax. Now try to blow raspberries with your lips – if you are having problems with that, then hum. The aim is for your lips to tingle; if they do, you will have successfully released all your throat, neck and diaphragm muscles, to allow good, clear, strong speech.

Stretch 3: Eyebrow raise

Raise your eyebrows to the ceiling and release them. This helps to release facial tension.

Stretch 4: Shoulder roll

Breathe in and roll your shoulders backwards, opening your chest; breathe out and let go. Make it as wide as you can across your chest with the least effort and without letting your shoulders rise up, and don't forget to breathe. This stretch releases your neck and chest muscles.

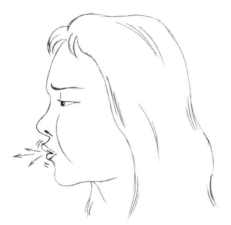

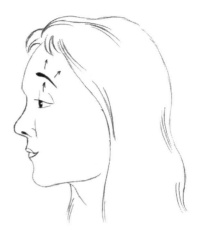

Stretch 2: releasing throat, neck and diaphragm muscles

Stretch 3: releasing facial tension

The following three exercise routines are useful to maintain flexibility and mobility in the upper body. See page 87 for an explanation of how to 'chin tuck'.

Exercise 1

Chin tuck then roll your shoulders backwards. Breathe in, grasping your hands together at the back of your chair at the same time as pulling your shoulder blades together. Breathe out.

Exercise 2

While seated, chin tuck then roll your shoulders backwards. Breathe in, stretching your arms above your head and reaching upwards, and breathe out at the top of the stretch.

Exercise 3

Chin tuck then do a shoulder roll backwards; while still sitting in your chair rotate your trunk, keeping your legs facing forwards. Make sure your legs are relaxed by gently wiggling them. Then place both hands onto the back of the chair, stretching your trunk as you breathe out. Return to the front and repeat, rotating to the other side.

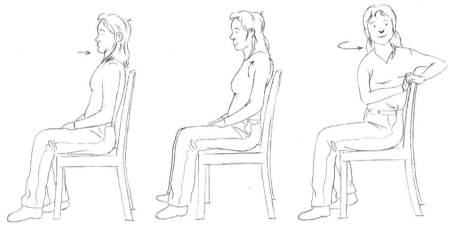

Chin tuck   Shoulder roll   Trunk rotation

Exercises for computer users and sedentary workers

Approximately every three minutes (occupational health and safety recommendations):

1. Stop, breathe out and drop your shoulders (but do not slouch).

2. Breathe in through your nose and belly.

3. Breathe out through your nose, release your shoulders and jaw, shake your hands.

The most important thing to do during a micropause break is to BREATHE OUT.

Chair exercises

The following chair exercises are for:

- relaxation of upper chest and neck muscles,
- stretching and mobilisation of the chest and neck muscles,
- general mobilising.

Neck nimbler

While seated, breathe out; let your chin come forward onto your chest, breathe in and out then relax; return to a normal position. Repeat this three times.

Shoulder roller

Breathe in; roll your shoulders backwards and let go. Repeat three times. Place your hands on top of your shoulders, breathe out and make circular, clockwise movements with your elbows.

Trunk twister

Keeping your hands on your shoulders, this time rotate your body to the left then the right. Repeat six times.

Back bender

This time breathe in and lift your arms above your head; breathe out and stretch backwards.

Leg lifter

Lift your knees up and down alternately until they feel tired and slightly achy.

Additional exercises to do in pairs

The two following exercises are excellent for muscular health, spinal mobility and general wellbeing. They are fantastic for relaxation and only need to be done for a couple of minutes to be effective. Both exercises are helpful during and after an episode of asthma as they encourage relaxation and exhalation.

The Breathing Works walk

While one person is sitting, the other locates their spine; the area to be worked on is from the base of the neck to approximately just below the shoulder blades. With first and second fingers start 'walking' up and down either side of the spine (nice and close to the spinal vertebrae), next to the spinal bump, using firm pressure.

The Breathing Works rock

With the person still sitting, place one hand on the front of their chest. Maintain pressure so the body does not move, and using your thumb and first finger locate the spinal bump called the spinous process. Firmly place your finger and thumb over each side of the vertebrae and oscillate gently back and forth from side to side for approximately 30 seconds on each vertebra, working down to shoulder blade level and back again. This is deliciously relaxing.

Trigger-point therapy

Through overuse, upper body muscles can become sore, tight and painful, resulting in very tender spots; these areas are commonly called trigger-points. The most common trigger-points can be found in the upper trapezius. When you have found the position shown in the picture place a reasonable amount of pressure on the spot; hold. You can wiggle the point if you wish for 30 seconds; repeat until tenderness fades. Follow this with three shoulder rolls backwards.

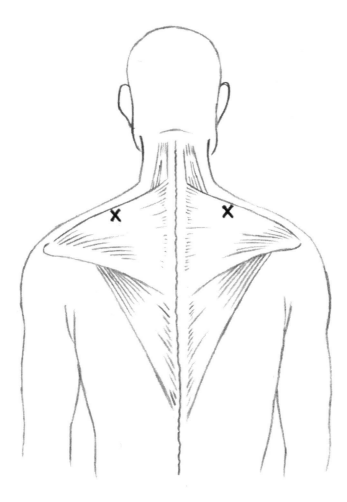

CHAPTER 11

Allergies

An allergy is a reaction to exposure to a specific substance called an allergen. An allergy occurs when our body perceives something to be life-threatening when in reality it should not be. For example, eating a peanut, exposure to grass pollen or getting a bee sting. The immune system kicks into action like an army going into battle and full-blown war results: if we get eczema our skin breaks out in welts, if we get hay fever our nose will stream, and if we get asthma our lungs tighten. All in all it is not a pleasant experience.

The process starts with sensitisation. The immune system comes into contact with a particular allergen, say a pollen, this is then committed to memory and the body produces specific antibodies (IgE) against it. With time and further exposure to the pollen (the allergen) the body continues the process until finally an allergic response occurs. The period of sensitisation can take weeks to years; for instance, in the case of pollen allergies it takes a number of seasons for the body to become sensitised to the pollen, therefore taking several years before an allergic reaction occurs.

Allergies tend to be inherited. In asthma the main allergens tend to be pollen, dust mites, animals with fur or feathers, and moulds – food tends to be not so common. Allergies are a major contributing cause for asthma; it is believed that up to 80 per cent of children with asthma have allergies.

I had never heard of the allergic march until my son James was experiencing it. It all started with a food allergy at seven months. We had returned from a walk on a hot summer's day. James was ready for his dinner and I was parched from the heat, so whilst feeding him I was helping myself to a bowl of ice-cream using the same spoon; halfway through his meal I noticed he started to cough, he then started to go limp, his breathing became laboured, his lips started to swell and his skin colour changed. Something was wrong and seriously wrong. I flung open the double doors and screamed to my neighbour who had toddlers herself; she arrived and immediately rang 999 – James was having an anaphylactic reaction. It took some time before we put two and two together, realising that James had a milk allergy and the residue on the spoon from the ice-cream was enough to cause this reaction. Milk allergies are very common. James then went on to develop mild eczema. We were breathing a sigh of relief as things started to settle down when asthma hit at two years old. I was devastated. This took us along another path of specialists and here I learnt of the allergic march. James grew out of the asthma at age five to finally develop allergic rhinitis at seven, which will apparently be permanent.

I am told that James has the classic march – this is where each organ becomes susceptible to sensitivities at some stage: the gut leading to food allergies, skin leading to eczema, lungs leading to asthma, and nose leading to allergic rhinitis. The march is something you cannot stop, but you can help to reduce the sensitivity to allergens. One way of doing this is by avoiding over-exposure to potential allergens that will cause a reaction. The most common food culprits are cow's milk and dairy products, nuts, wheat, food additives, eggs and shellfish. Other factors are dust mites, moulds and pollens.

A family history of allergies is often an indicator since there is a strong genetic factor; in our case my husband had severe asthma as a child and a family history of allergies. Try to avoid antibiotics early on, it is often better to fight the infection and build up immunity (this, of course, within reason). Also, research is now finding we are too clean and by sterilising our surfaces with strong cleaning agents could be eliminating helpful germs. Cleanliness is very important but let children explore. Visit the allergy awareness websites and find out what to avoid when breast feeding or during pregnancy. Once you know your child has an allergy, awareness of other factors helps. In James' case I did everything to avoid allergen exposure – for dust mites we had wooden floors, protective bedding, frequent cleaning, and no cats: apparently even if you do not have a cat, the cat hair from others in preschool can be enough to increase sensitisation. Baby number two is nearly here and I have to the best of my ability followed the guidelines of things to avoid. Crossing fingers.

Natalie, mother of James, 8

It is known that infants with eczema have a greater chance of getting hay fever or asthma by preschool age. Paediatricians in Sweden studied 94 children with eczema from infancy to the age of seven and the results of the study showed that the eczema improved in 82 of the children. However, 43 per cent developed asthma and 45 per cent developed hay fever.

Eczema in infants is usually triggered by foods, especially cow's milk. Hay fever and asthma in school children is usually triggered by airborne allergens, such as dust mites. This change in allergy from babies to older children is called the 'allergic march'.

Are allergies the cause of asthma?

Identification of allergies is not always easy; the best route is to visit an allergist. However, not all of us are able to do this. The next best thing is to work from checklists: record dates, times, activities, peak flow rates and the severity of episodes. Make the list as detailed as possible.

Of course, with some allergies the reaction is obvious because they occur immediately, e.g. symptoms after sniffing a flower or after exposure to cats or wearing that jersey from last winter that has been sitting in a mouldy wardrobe. In true food allergies reactions occur very promptly and are often easy to diagnose: lips start to tingle and the mouth develops an odd numb sensation.

Some individuals are allergic to food additives; these can be hidden in many manufactured foods. Food intolerances will cause a reaction, however they do not involve the immune response associated with true food allergies. The reaction is often delayed and harder to diagnose. Investigation in the form of elimination diets is the best procedure with food intolerances.

Allergens affect us in different ways

Allergens that enter via the nose lead to hay fever, rhinitis and sinusitis; those that enter through the eye cause itchy, tearing eyes (conjunctivitis); through the voice box cause laryngitis, hoarseness and coughing; through the windpipe cause tracheitis; through the bronchial tubes, wheezing and coughing leading to asthma or bronchitis; and through the skin, contact dermatitis or eczema.

It is believed that the allergies are the baseline cause, not just a trigger: therefore reducing exposure is very important. This is possible once you have worked out the possible allergy.

The common allergens are dust mites, moulds, fungi, pollen, animal hair/fur, plants and cockroaches. Less common are latex, antibiotics, wool, cotton, other textiles, henna or allergens at work, e.g. sawdust, dust from soybeans.

There is a lot of literature on this topic, so please see the recommended reading list on page 110.

Note: Food intolerance or sensitivity accounts for only a small proportion of those with asthma.

The reaction

Exposure to allergens causes a chain reaction at cellular levels; as we have seen, it is like the body going into battle as the immune system attacks the allergen. Specialised cells release chemicals known as mediators, one of the best-known mediators being histamine. Histamine receptors in the lungs trigger contraction of the muscles of the bronchial tubes, causing broncho-spasm: this is the basic, underlying mechanism of asthma.

The effect of breathing on the allergic response

When we over-breathe this lowers the levels of carbon dioxide in the blood (hyperventilation); as a result this causes mast cells to release histamine more easily – in fact it leads to an excessive production of histamine. This in turn causes our airways to constrict, resulting in asthma. This highlights the vital importance of good breathing practices for people with allergies.

People with allergies often have many episodes of upper respiratory tract infections, hay fever, viral infections and common colds. Good breathing and nasal hygiene are essential to keep the immune system strong and the body healthy.

Factors that can assist in the allergic person

- Try to detect your allergen. If allergies are prevalent it is of vital importance to reduce the allergic response by reducing exposure to your allergen.
- Stay healthy, as when you are run-down and tired you are more susceptible to reacting to whatever your allergy is.
- Take medications as prescribed.
- Breathe well to maintain health and a strong immune system, and to avoid over-production of histamine.
- Exercise for the above reasons.
- Keep up to date with information on reduction of allergen exposure. (See page 111 for Allergy Awareness website details.)

Medications for asthma

For more information, advice and factsheets, contact the National Asthma Campaign. The information here should not replace the advice of a doctor.

Medications are useful because they can:
- remove symptoms, allowing you to exercise again, comfortably
- subdue the allergic reaction of your body and reduce the inflammation in the airways
- remove or lessen damaging effects on your lungs.

Which medication should be chosen?

Medicines for asthma are generally thought of in two main groups:
- Relievers (bronchodilators): these are quick-acting drugs that relax the muscles of the airways. They relieve the symptoms of wheeze, cough and breathlessness.
- Preventers: these act over a longer time and work by reducing the swelling and inflammation within the airways.

Relievers

There are three groups of these. All three types of reliever can be combined if necessary.

Beta$_2$-agonists

These drugs act on tiny receptors on the muscles of the bronchioles. The drug fits the receptor like a key fits a lock and stimulates the muscle to relax. Examples of those that act for a short time (three or four hours following a single dose) are salbutamol and terbutaline.

These drugs (and the other inhaled drugs below) are inhaled from a variety of delivery devices, the most familiar being the pressurised metered-dose-inhaler (MDI). Special adaptors and types of inhaler are available to make it easier to administer inhaled medication, especially to young children and the very elderly. Your doctor or practice nurse can recommend which type will be the most suitable.

Longer-acting beta$_2$-agonists include salmeterol. Their action lasts over twelve hours, making them suitable for twice-daily dosage. These medications are particularly good for exercise-induced problems and night-time symptoms.

Anticholinergics

One of the ways in which the size of the airways is naturally controlled is through nerves that connect to the muscles. The nerve impulses cause the muscles to contract, narrowing and tightening the airways. Anticholinergic drugs block this effect, allowing the airway to open. The size of this effect is fairly small, so it is most noticeable if the airways have already been narrowed by other conditions, such as chronic bronchitis. These drugs are therefore not commonly used in children, but ipratropium is available for use in children if required.

Preventers

The following medications are given by mouth and are more likely to give side-effects than inhaled treatments. They may cause a racing heart, restlessness and difficulty sleeping. They are still in very wide use throughout the world.

There are three main groups:

Corticosteroids

Corticosteroids (or steroids e.g. beclomethasone and fluticosone) have made an enormous difference to the management of asthma. They work to reduce the amount of inflammation and swelling within the airways, reducing their tendency to contract, and have allowed many people with previously troublesome asthma to lead almost symptom-free lives, although sometimes short courses of oral steroid tablets may be required for bad attacks. Although steroids are powerful drugs with many potential side-effects, their safety in asthma has been well established. It is also important to balance the problems that arise from poorly treated asthma against the improvement in health that occurs when the condition is well treated.

Cromones

There are two drugs in this group: sodium cromoglycate and nedocromil. They also act to reduce airway inflammation. They tend to be best for mild asthma and are more effective in children as a first-line preventative treatment, but may take up to six weeks to have an effect and are rarely used in the UK.

Leukotriene receptor antagonists

Leukotrienes are compounds released by inflammatory cells within the lung and have a constricting effect upon the airways. By blocking this effect with these antagonist drugs the constriction is reversed. Montelukast and Zafirlukast are presently licensed for children and adults in the UK to treat mild to moderate asthma that is not adequately controlled with inhalers.

   As with any medication – make sure you know exactly what it is and why you are using it. Ask questions and make sure you understand fully.

Reinforcement of upper chest breathing patterns is commonly caused by the misuse of inhalers – the rapid upper chest heave to inhale the medication. Check your inhaler technique (see page 102).

Inhalers

Next time you use your inhaler check the way you inhale. Watch yourself in the mirror – and watch your upper chest. Avoid reinforcing upper chest patterns by learning to inhale abdominally when you use your inhaler.

- Before using your inhaler, practise inhaling by leading with the diaphragm.
- Take a strong mouth-breath in with slightly pursed lips.
- Try this with your hands clasped behind your head.
- Feel your stomach expand as you inhale.

It's very easy to slip back into old patterns, especially if these have become ingrained. Some doctors even think that bad inhaler techniques may actually trigger hyperventilation or asthma. Make sure you get it right so that the medications can work their wonders with the minimum dosage.

Puffers and other devices

It makes good sense to breathe asthma medicines straight into your lungs. If you can use the direct route, you only need a small dose of medicine and it will start working quickly. Any medicine you swallow goes the long way round to your lungs. This takes time and some gets lost on the journey, so you need to take a higher dose and allow extra time for it to start working.

Why so many different inhalers?

Different drug companies make products in each group and they come in different strengths and forms. Asthma medicines can be divided into two groups: preventers and relievers. One group (mainly brown, also red or orange inhalers) helps prevent the swelling and narrowing inside the airways and is used every day. The other group (mainly blue inhalers) relieves symptoms by relaxing tightened muscles surrounding the airways.

How do you choose?

The choices are between aerosol and powder inhalers. You should have a device that you feel is easy to use.

Aerosol inhalers

The medicine and a liquid propellant are forced under pressure into a small canister, which is put into the coloured plastic case. When the inhaler is pressed, a measured dose of medicine is released through the mouthpiece. Exactly the same dose is released each time. It is important to shake the inhaler vigorously before each puff so you mix up the medicine and propellant evenly. It comes out very fast and needs to be breathed in carefully so it gets deep into the lungs, not just all around the mouth. Always keep a spare inhaler in reserve.

What else should we know about aerosol inhalers?

- They are cheap, convenient and come in a variety of strengths.
- They can be used with a variety of spacer devices (explained below), which can often improve their performance.
- Most inhalers have 200 doses, although some have 112, 120 or 400 doses.
- All aerosol inhalers use propellants, although the amount involved is small. Non-CFC propellants are now becoming available.
- Some brown, red or orange inhalers (preventers) may cause hoarseness or thrush in the mouth. Gargling with water (and spitting out afterwards) and using the inhaler with a spacer usually solves this problem.
- Some common mistakes are:
  - not shaking the inhaler well enough
  - breathing out too hard so you cough

- pressing the puffer TOO EARLY before you have started to breathe in (see the mist!)
- breathing in TOO FAST.

How to look after your aerosol inhaler

- Your inhaler can get clogged, especially where the medicine sprays out. To clean it, remove the canister, wash the plastic case in soapy water, rinse and leave to dry.
- Always keep the cap on your inhaler when it's not in use, to keep it clean.
- Don't store spare inhalers in a hot place, such as a car glovebox.

How to use your inhaler

1. Shake your inhaler vigorously. Take off the cap and hold the inhaler upright. Shaking the medication evenly and holding it upright means you will get a full dose.

2. Sit upright and tilt your head back. Tilting your head back opens your throat.

3. Breathe out with a sigh. By doing this you can take more in when you puff the inhaler.

4. Hold the inhaler upright and close your mouth around the mouthpiece.

5. Breathe in slowly and deeply, pressing your inhaler once just after you begin to breathe in. A slow inhalation gets the medicine right down into your lungs.

6. Hold your breath for 10 seconds if possible. The medication is a very fine powder and holding your breath gives it more time to settle in your lungs.

7. Breathe out gently through your nose.

When to start a new inhaler

Always have a spare inhaler ready and start this before the old one is completely empty. There are extra doses in every aerosol but these may not have the correct mixture of medicine and propellant. When you shake the inhaler you will still hear the propellant, even though the medicine has run out. So although you may 'hear' medicine, it may not come out or may not seem to work.

Start the new inhaler once the 60/112/200/400 doses (number of doses is indicated on the inhaler) have been taken. This will be before the inhaler is completely empty.

You will be aware if a reliever medicine is no longer working, but with a preventer there is not an immediate change to warn you that the inhaler should be discarded. It may help to write the start date on the preventer inhaler.

The autohaler

The autohaler is an aerosol inhaler but contains less propellant because it is breath activated. You lift a small lever before shaking, to prepare the metered dose for release. Breathe out, place the inhaler in your mouth and breathe in. This releases the dose. At first, it may take a little practice to continue breathing in once the dose is released.

The autohaler overcomes the problem of trying to press the inhaler and breathe in at exactly the right time. It is available as a preventer in two different strengths and as a reliever. (The reliever contains 400 doses.)

Spacer devices

Spacers are specially designed tubes. You put a puff of asthma medicine from your aerosol inhaler into it and then breathe in through a mouthpiece or use a mask.

How does it help?

- It makes aerosol inhalers easier to use, more effective, and reduces side-effects.
- It is suitable for all ages. Spacers with masks are designed to help very young children take their medication correctly.
- You get 50 per cent more medicine into your lungs than you could just using your inhaler on its own.
- It slows down the speed of the aerosol so less medicine gets left in the mouth and throat.
- It reduces the chance of hoarseness and thrush in your mouth from preventer medicine.
- It helps when you are short of breath and an inhaler is difficult to use.
- It is a convenient compact alternative to a nebuliser (see page 107). Studies on adults and children show spacers work just as well as nebulisers in acute asthma.

Cleaning a spacer

Priming

Because a static charge builds up inside the spacer it must be 'primed' before first use. Wash it in hot water plus liquid detergent. Do not rinse, as detergent helps to reduce the static charge. Leave to drip dry. Rinsing with water and rubbing the spacer dry can increase the static, which attracts the medicine to the sides of the spacer, meaning you get much less in your lungs. If the spacer is only used occasionally, it will need washing again before use.

Regular cleaning

Wash in soapy water (as for priming) every week or more often if using Intal or Tilade. A sticky valve and powder build-up makes the spacer less effective. Follow the manufacturer's instructions if the spacer is to be taken apart for cleaning.

How to use your spacer

Only ever put ONE PUFF of your medicine in the spacer at a time. Remove and shake the inhaler before the next puff. If you put in more than one puff the droplets of spray join together and won't go as far down into the lungs, so you actually receive less medication.

1. Fit the mask (if necessary).
2. Shake the inhaler well (holding it upright).
3. Fit the inhaler into the opening at the end of the spacer.
4. Seal lips firmly round the mouthpiece or place the mask so that it seals around the nose and mouth.
5. Press the inhaler once then take a slow deep breath through the mouth and hold your breath for up to 10 seconds.
6. Breathe out slowly.
7. If very breathless, deep breaths are impossible. Instead take 2-3 (adult) or 5-6 (child) smaller slow breaths, keeping the spacer in the mouth or the mask firmly fixed all the time.
8. Repeat steps 2 to 7 for each dose of medicine.

What else should we know about spacers?

There are large and small spacers available. The Volumatic and Nebuhaler are examples of large spacers made for particular brands of inhalers. The Aerochamber and Able Spacer are smaller and have flexible fittings that take any aerosol inhaler. Masks can be fitted over the mouthpiece of some spacers. Others have fixed masks.

Points to remember:
- Use your spacer with any aerosol inhaler, preventer or reliever.
- It cannot be used with powder inhalers (Turbohaler, Diskhaler) or Autohaler.
- A valve in the spacer mouthpiece end opens as you breathe in (an adult should check that the valve moves with young children) and closes as you breathe out.
- With large-volume spacers, tilt the spacer upwards at a 45 degree angle. This helps the valve work best. If a mask is used it must fit the face firmly or the spacer valve won't work. When using a spacer and mask with a brown, red or orange inhaled steroid (preventer), wipe the face afterwards to remove any traces of medicine. Otherwise just rinse the mouth with water, gargle and spit out after using preventer medicine.
- Start breathing from the spacer as soon as possible after pressing the inhaler. Keep the inhaler steady – shaking it about will make the spray particles join together.
- Spacers can be obtained on prescription or they can be purchased from a pharmacy.

Dry powder inhalers

Accuhaler

This is used for relievers and preventers. Doses of the medicine are set into a foil strip. There is a dose counter. The case is opened to reveal a lever, which activates the dose. The medicine is taken by breathing in through the mouthpiece. You must not breathe back into the Accuhaler. There are no propellants involved; it may take two breaths to get the full dose.

Diskhaler

This is used for relievers and preventers. Doses of the medicine are set into a circular foil disk. The lid of the Diskhaler is lifted to puncture a dose. The medicine is taken by breathing in through the mouthpiece. You must not breathe back into the Diskhaler.

Points to remember:
- There are no propellants involved, so it may take two breaths to get the full dose.
- The lid must be pulled vertical to pierce the blister.
- The Diskhaler is reloaded when empty.
- It is easy to check how many doses have been used, although the Diskhaler may be fiddly for the elderly and those with hand problems.
- Separate Diskhalers should be used for relievers and preventers.
- Use the brush provided to clean up the loose powder when the disk is changed.

Turbohaler

The Turbohaler comes in reliever, preventer and combination canisters. They are easily identified by their colour bases – blue for reliever, brown for preventer and red for combination. Each Turbohaler holds 200 prepacked doses of medicine. Twisting the grip at the base one way and then back again while holding the device upright makes it ready to use. The dose is breathed in strongly and steadily through the mouthpiece.

Further points:
- The Turbohaler has no propellant or filler added to the medicine. This means you will hardly notice any powder in your mouth.
- When a red tape shows at the top of the small window only 20 doses remain. (The powder you can hear when you shake the Turbohaler is a drying agent, not the medicine.)
- A deep steady inhalation is needed to use the Turbohaler, but breath-holding afterwards is not required.
- A special base can be attached to the base of the Turbohaler to make it easier to grip for people with hand disabilities.

How to clean the Turbohaler

Remove the mouthpiece and clean at least weekly. Wipe any particles which have stuck underneath using a dry cloth. Do not wash the mouthpiece. *Keep the cap on when not in use.*

Combination

A new red inhaler which combines a long-acting 'reliever' (beta$_2$-agonist) and an inhaled steroid 'preventer' (corticosteroids) in one device is available under certain conditions.

Nebulisers

These are an alternative device for taking medication. Nebulisers produce a fine mist of the medicine and are powered by either an electrical air pump or oxygen. It takes about 10 minutes to breathe in the dose. A nebuliser is only suitable for certain circumstances. It is mainly used for reliever medicine but can be used for some preventers for very young children, although the alternative of a spacer with a mask may be better. With so many improved devices and spacers, there is less need for nebulisers.

Summary

Inhalers are an important part of asthma care. Many people dislike using medicines, but used correctly asthma medicines are very safe, even for small children and pregnant women. Inhaled medicines are best as they work quickly and require only small amounts of drug. And because inhalers come in many different shapes and sizes, it's easy to find one that suits you best.

Other co-existing breathing disorders

Asthma is known as a 'reversible obstructive' disorder. 'Obstructive' because airways can become clogged with mucus from the swelling of your airways, and reversible because the symptoms can reverse either spontaneously or with treatment. Sometimes people with asthma have other obstructive disorders as well, which are known by a variety of names:

- COPD (Chronic Obstructive Pulmonary Disease)
- CORD (Chronic Obstructive Respiratory Disease)
- COAD (Chronic Obstructive Airways Disease)

and the much snappier title which leaves out the word 'disease' –

- CAL (Chronic Airway Limitation)

These titles usually refer to chronic bronchitis and emphysema which can often overlap with asthma as well, particularly if you've been a smoker or have lived and/or worked in a heavily polluted environment.

Although the breathlessness of an asthma attack can be relieved by the use of 'reliever' puffers, the breathlessness of CAL may be less responsive because of permanent airways and air sac damage. This can be frightening and uncomfortable and lead to your becoming less active. Because it seems easier to upper chest mouth-breathe this 'bad' pattern is likely to become a 'bad' habit.

The same problems strike as in asthma:

- upper chest-breathing patterns (so costly of energy, see page 37)
- ineffective coughing
- giving exercise a wide berth, leading to loss of fitness
- stress and anxiety.

The breathing and coughing advice in this book will be of benefit to you. But other things are imperative as well:

- Improve your muscle strength.
- Stop smoking.
- Feeling breathless is a sign to stop and recover: STOP DROP FLOP (see page 60). But it's not harmful to be breathless.
- Keep your diaphragm pattern strong as well as strengthening the rest of your body.
- Practise relaxing your upper chest muscles while you're sitting or lying.
- Using Rest Positions (see page 38) when you feel breathless helps recovery.
- IMT (described on page 58) may be very helpful in mild to moderate cases – not to mention enjoyable! It's a positive way to desensitise yourself to fear of breathlessness as well as strengthening your inspiratory muscles. (It's not advisable in severe cases because of the danger of overloading very weakened muscles.)
- Improve fitness levels. Asthma Societies as well as most hospital physiotherapy departments run excellent courses where you can be assessed and regain confidence by exercising in a safe environment.

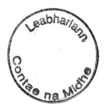

Useful resources

Asthma information on the Internet

UK National Asthma Campaign: www.asthma.org.uk

British Allergy Foundation: www.allergyfoundation.com

American Academy of Allergy Asthma and Immunology: www.aaaai.org

Canadian Asthma Society: www.asthma.ca

National Asthma Council, Australia: nationalasthma.org.au

Asthma Australia: www.asthmaaustralia.org.au

Asthma and Respiratory Foundation of New Zealand: www.asthmanz.co.nz

Other helpful sites

www.dhd.com (for information on the Acapella® positive expiratory pressure device)

www.breathingworks.com

www.powerbreathe.com (for information on inspiratory muscle training devices)

Recommended reading

Brookes, T. *Catching my breath: an asthmatic explores his illness*.
Vintage Books, 1992.

Brostoff, J & Gamlin, L. *Asthma: the complete guide*.
Bloomsbury, London, 1999.

Asthma and allergy support organizations

Allergy UK (formerly known as British Allergy Foundation)

Deepdene House · 30 Bellegrove Road · Welling · Kent · DA16 3PY

Tel: 020 8303 8525

Helpline: 020 8303 8583 (9am–9pm Mon–Fri, 10am–1pm Sat)

www.allergyfoundation.com

Useful website with information about allergies and allergy testing. The foundation offers information, advice and support to allergy sufferers and their carers and raises funds for allergy research .

British Lung Foundation

78 Hatton Garden · London · EC1B 1PX

Tel: 020 7831 5831

www.lunguk.org

Charity funding new research into lung diseases. Offers support to those affected with the disease, and provides information on lung disease and lung health. Website gives information on research and has fact sheet on asthma.

National Asthma Campaign (NAC)

Providence House · Providence Place · London · N1 0NT

Tel: 020 7226 2260

Helpline: 0845 7 01 02 03 (9am–7pm Mon–Fri)

www.asthma.org.uk

The NAC campaigns for the interests of people with asthma, provides public information in the form of leaflets and other publications and funds research. Its website contains up-to-the minute news and information for anyone affected by asthma. Its helpline takes over 18,000 calls a year.

National Asthma Campaign Scotland

2a North Charlotte Street · Edinburgh · EH2 4HR

Tel: 0131 226 2544

National Society for Research into Allergies

PO Box 45 · Hinckley · Leicestershire · LE10 1JY

Tel: 01455 851546

A charity founded in 1979, it offers practical, constructive advice and support to affected persons, carers and medical professionals, and links to others where possible. Activities include funding research and raising awareness of allergy and environmental diseases.

Asthma Society of Ireland

Eden House · 15–17 Eden Quay · Dublin 1

Tel: 01 878 8511

Helpline: 1850 44 54 64 (24 hours a day, 7 days a week)

asthma@indigo.ie

www.asthmasociety.ie

Provides information, advice and reassurance to people with asthma and their families. Works to promote awareness and understanding of the condition among the general public.

Asthma Society of Canada

130 Bridgeland Avenue · Suite 425 · Toronto · Ontario · M6A 1Z4

Tel: 1-800-787-3880 Toll Free

Tel: 416 787-4050 Local (for Toronto residents)

info@asthma.ca

www.asthma.ca

The Asthma and Respiratory Foundation of New Zealand Inc.

Rossmore House · 123 Moleworth Street · PO Box 1459 · Wellington

www.asthmanz.co.nz

Index

Emergency strategies

Assess

Mild? Short of breath, wheeze, cough, chest tightness.

Moderate? Loud wheeze, breathing difficulty, can only speak in short sentences.

Severe? Distressed, gasping for breath, difficulty speaking two words, blueness around the mouth.

If the person has severe asthma or is frightened, call an ambulance IMMEDIATELY – DIAL 999.

Sit

Sit the person upright in a Rest Position (see page 38) and stay with them. Reassure calmly.

Treat

Treat with 6 puffs of a blue 'reliever' inhaler.

Use a spacer for aerosol inhaler if available. (One puff at a time in the spacer, person to take 6 breaths.)

Help

If not improving after 6 minutes, **call the ambulance**. Continue to use the blue inhaler, 6 puffs (as above) every 6 minutes until help arrives.

In this situation you will not overdose the person by giving them the reliever every 6 minutes.

Monitor

If improving after 6 minutes, keep monitoring. If necessary repeat doses of blue inhaler.

All OK!

When free of wheeze, cough and breathlessness, return to normal **quiet** activity. If symptoms recur, repeat treatment and rest. See your doctor.